Can't Stop the Sunrise

Adventures in Healing Confronting Corruption & the Journey to Institutional Reform

by

Vanessa Osage

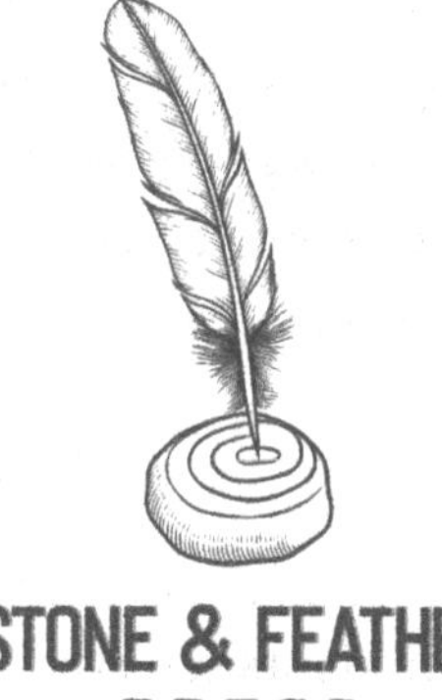

STONE & FEATHER PRESS
·WASHINGTON, USA·

Stone & Feather Press
publishes stories that may otherwise be forgotten.
We advance human, civil, and environmental rights
by promoting justice through powerful storytelling.

Published by Stone & Feather Press
Washington, United States of America
www.stoneandfeatherpress.com

ISBN 978-1-7356082-0-4 pbk.
ISBN 978-1-7356082-1-1 h.c.

Printed in the United States of America
Set in Hoefler Text & Helvetica
Cover Design by Booklerk
Hand Lettering by Natalia Mikhaleva
Ink Drawings by Mehvina Naeem

This book is dedicated to
everyone who speaks the truth,
even when it's hard.

The Amends Project is a Washington state nonprofit with a mission to "mend the loophole that has allowed for the cover-up of child abuse at independent schools: implementing The Justice CORPS Initiative."

It was officially established in 2019 to bring transparency to New England boarding schools and private institutions across the country.

Yet the story began much earlier . . .

Goals of The Amends Project

Bring the truth to light
Hold leaders accountable
Enact lasting, positive change

~ Chapters ~

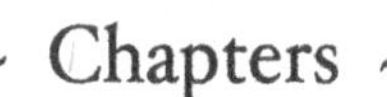

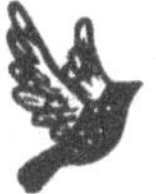

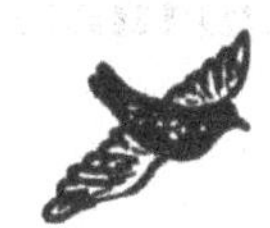

Welcome

Introduction 1

Character Reference . . . 5

Origins

Flying Toward a New Dawn . . . 8

Roots 10

The Stories We Tell ~
In the Beginning 16

On Education 20

Dethroning ~
the Seat of Authority 25

Major Blessing ~
Friendship 29

The Door Through
Which You Came,
The First Door 33

Nearly Ran Away 38

Useful Skills ~
Not Caring
What People Think 43

The Door Through
Which You Came,
The Second Door 47

Departures

On the Road 56

The Body Speaks, 2001 68

Ask & You Shall Receive, Part One 73

Trauma - The Live Wire of Survival 76

Useful Skills - Willing to Piss People Off 80

Already on My Way 83

The Speech 87

Waves of Reckoning 96

Belonging - A Home in One's Heart 101

Major Blessing - Chosen Coping Strategy 104

The Body Speaks, 2005 . . . 108

Arrivals 120

Encounters

Major Blessing - My First Love 125

Definitions 129

On the Whys & Recovery . 130

Useful Skills - Watch What People Do 132

Tactics - D Words 134

Apocalypse - The Unveiling 136

Checking In 140

Ask & You Shall Receive, Part Two 142

Intentions - The Amends Project 147

Crossroads & Divergences . 152

Integration, East & West 155

Quick, She's Coming! 166

Paradigms Collide 192

Diminishing - Stay Appropriate Size 182

Go On, Tell Me to Be Quiet Again! 184

The Feature Article, The Lowell Sun 193

Still They Came - Waking Up 197

We Are With You 205

Falling & Rising 209

A Breather for Healing . . 218

Diversion - Stay Focused . 222

Warriors of Presence 223

The Double-Talk Shuffle 234

Discrediting & Defamation - Be Who You Are 230

Oversight - This is for Everyone . . . 248

Destruction & Rebirth . . 242

On the Culture of a Place. 254

All Survivors Day 260

Returns

Open House 264

Balancing That Story . . . 282

Their Report & Mine . . . 289

Would Never = Hasn't Yet 309

Stories We Tell -

Misleading Public Statements 312

Who Can We Tell? 317

On Apology 330

I Decline Your Offer As It Stands 338

White Male Privilege: Q & A 356

Useful Skills - Staying With It 368

Major Blessing - The Many Gratitudes . 380

Ancient Parable 391

Value & Appreciation . . 393

Intersections - Internal Biases, External Consequences . 314

Justice CORPS Video . . 325

The Courage to Repair . . 336

Parent Letter 343

Wikipedia 346

Male Initiation - Humanizing 362

Lucid Dream Road 374

Taking Action - 2020 & Beyond 385

Choose Your Own Ending 392

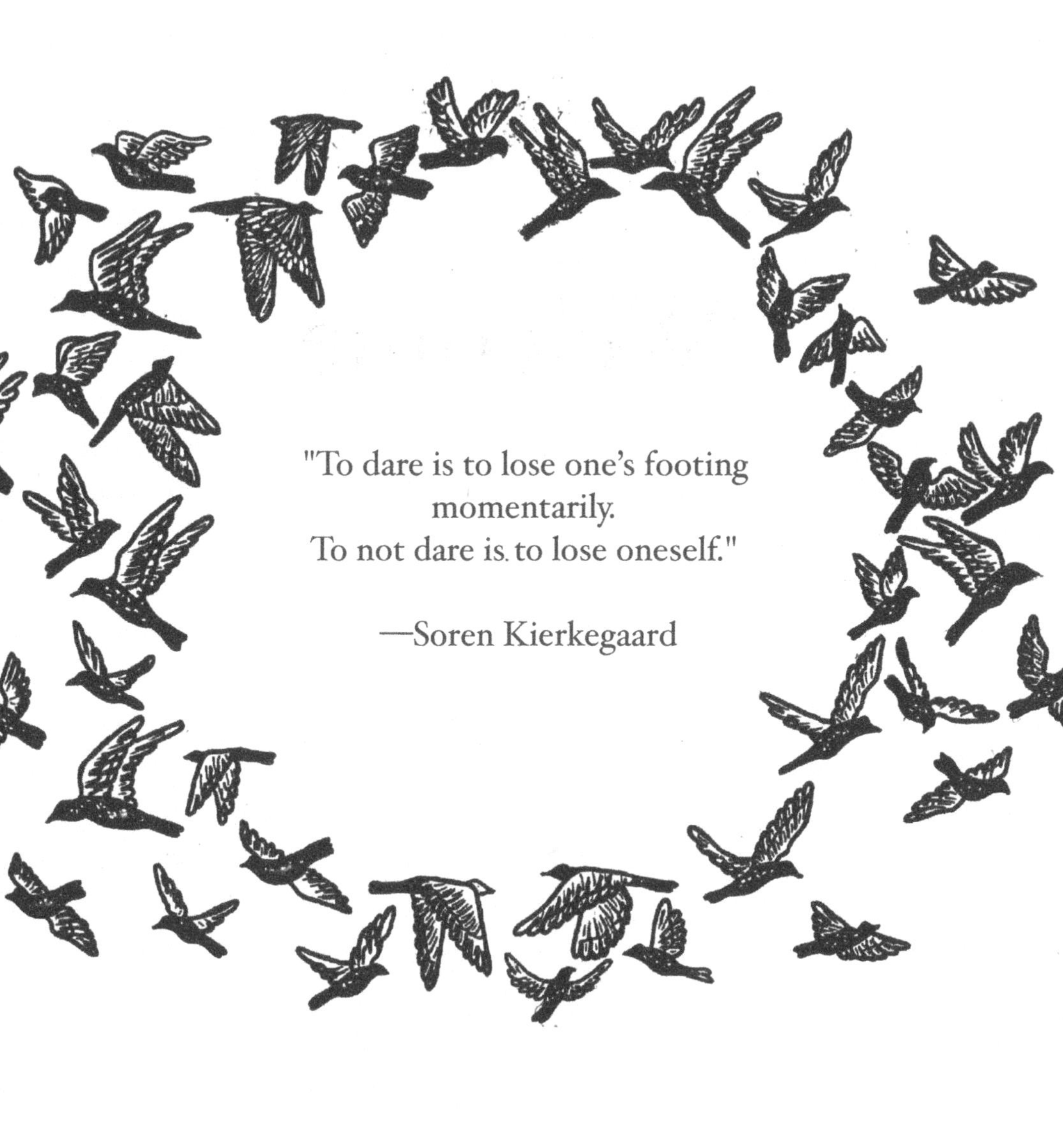

"To dare is to lose one's footing
momentarily.
To not dare is to lose oneself."

—Soren Kierkegaard

Welcome

This is a story that exists inside many stories. It calls to you from a new time, as the old story falls away, and our brightest collective vitality cries out for rebirth. It shows us who we are and who we might become, while revealing a world you may or may not recognize.

Because this is a story, in part, about the importance of calling out corruption - I will be naming names. I do this to protect the truth and not those who seek to silence it. I will add the requisite "alleged" where needed and report the stories as they were told to me. As my attorney friend says, the ultimate defense of libel is the truth.

Where peripheral characters are involved, I will use pseudonyms or remove identifying characteristics to protect their choice to live with anonymity. Exposure in our lives is always a personal decision. I will honor their choice in this way.

You will find a reference of names and characters following this introduction. Access to full news articles and editorials online may be found in the footnotes.

I will talk of understanding what it takes to speak truth to power and to keep speaking until you get the necessary results for the betterment of our world.

I also want to acknowledge that I am in possession of traits which I have not earned, yet have made my journey to influencing change all the more possible and successful. I want to own my privilege: I live the benefits of whiteness (even while ethnic-looking), I am a heterosexual, cis-gendered female and considered by some to be beautiful. This last piece was my first lived-experience of recognizing a 'privilege', *Because of this thing I can't take credit for, people treat me differently.* How risky it feels to even name it here! I will strive to honestly name the threads of injustice that weave throughout abuses of power.

So many people have shared their stories with me now, that I long to trace the web of ill health in its fullest picture, so we can begin to dismantle it. The intersection of many social and societal truths converge in these kinds of stories. These, when spoken clearly and honestly, I hope, are the truths that can save lives.

I also grew up - if precariously - among the advantages of financial wealth and excess. I am telling stories about private schools, elite institutions and the kinds of ills that have taken hold there. I am compelled to continue working in this realm (even as I do not live there) because so many of the 'decision-makers' of society have sprung from these places. Corrupt, elite high schools risk breeding corrupt, ivy-league college students, who are susceptible to becoming corrupt attorneys, politicians and/or decision-makers.

Unless, of course, we do something about it.

I am starting where I have been given an entry-point from which to make change. This book is about doing something about it.

I will name and identify my personal blessings - which arise in the course of a lifetime - and celebrate each one as we go. But, I must say humbly, I have been able to walk this particular road because I have not had to walk the challenges of others. This country has many an imbalance to address, many a horrific trespass against individuals and groups of people which disgrace our shared story as a nation. The necessary process of acknowledgement and reconciliation is long overdue. This work is just one contribution to the righting of so many injustices calling for repair and rebalance in our time. I walk into this story with you, holding that awareness.

From the cultural reckoning, I am striving to evoke the necessary actions of a response. In laying out all that has happened, I am outlining patterns that I hope will make us wiser and more equipped to enact positive change. I am reporting back, after hacking through much confusion on the daunting, painful, agonizing, and sometimes energizing and liberating path of confronting corruption. I have arrived somewhere new. I've walked through those brambles and emerge with a few threads of clarity, which I dearly hope will become lifelines to those traveling similar paths. I extend my hand now, to show you what remains after persisting and enduring for so long. *Here, I found a thread that connects to a place of light and truth. May I hand it to you?*

Perhaps you find yourself on a similar journey. Imbalances of power can arise on many levels: within one human heart, one intimate relationship, one family, one school, one religious organization, one nation or one world. From what I've seen to this point, the pattern is always the same. So, we each have infinite chances to restore a natural balance, right where we are.

Given that this is my story (and my inner punk-ass finds expression here), I will be swearing. I will only seek to do it well, and you may now consider yourself forewarned.

I also speak as a Certified Sexuality Educator (CSE, Planned Parenthood), with over a decade of experience teaching Comprehensive Sexuality Education to ages 4 & up. I have been a Consultant & Professional Coach to adults in emotional and sexual health for just as long. So, you will meet my love and fascination for the human heart, and the ways our bodies respond and evolve toward health.

Within all dark things, there is the potential for a lesson - and a new strength to help pull us through. I will name these skills as well, as beams of clarity that point the way to a solution. That is the eventual redemption of this story.

We will get there.

I write this piece during the first global pandemic in known history. Old and existing structures are breaking down, and many will need to be rebuilt. I hope these insights are timely (maybe even timeless), as we'll be asked to consider what new systems could better serve us going forward. I have a plan and a vision, informed by the story that has preceded it.

This is a story that exists inside many stories. Of power and resistance, of the deeply personal as it reaches the political and global experiences. It rides the rolling currents of social change, traversing interconnected waterways, and offers you what you will find.

It is a reflection, a guide and a call to action. This is my invitation to you, to see yourself in this story and to be moved where you will, to carry its message forward in your best possible way.

It is a reminder of what matters most and how that might be guarded and protected. It is a question for your consideration and contemplation, what matters most to you?

It is, for you, something that will be uniquely and only for you. In that, it is a mystery...

Welcome to the Beginning.

- Character Reference -

Lawrence Academy is a co-ed boarding high school in rural Groton, Massachusetts, thirty five miles northwest of Boston. Founded in 1792, the current annual tuition for a boarding student is $65,925/year.

Steven L Hahn was headmaster of Lawrence Academy from 1984 to 2002

Peter Regis, the groundskeeper from 1988 - 2001

Bruce MacNeil, Board of Trustees member from 1984 to present, recent President of the Board

Dan Scheibe (shy-bee) headmaster from 2012 to present

Libby Margraf, Assistant Headmaster (current)

Paul Lannon, of Holland & Knight Law Firm, attorney for the school, from 2001 to present

Jamie Baker, (former) Assistant Headmaster for Academics, from 2018-2019

Mitchell Garabedian, Boston-area attorney, specializing in institutional sexual abuse cases since 1979

The Lowell Sun, regional newspaper to the greater Boston, Lowell, Massachusetts and New Hampshire area since 1878

Rick Sobey, Lowell Sun reporter who first picked up the story in 2018

Jim Campinini, editor of The Lowell Sun until 2018

Tom Zuppa, editor of The Sun from December 2018 - April 2019

Origins

"And suddenly you know:
It's time to start something new
and trust the magic of beginnings."

— Meister Eckhart

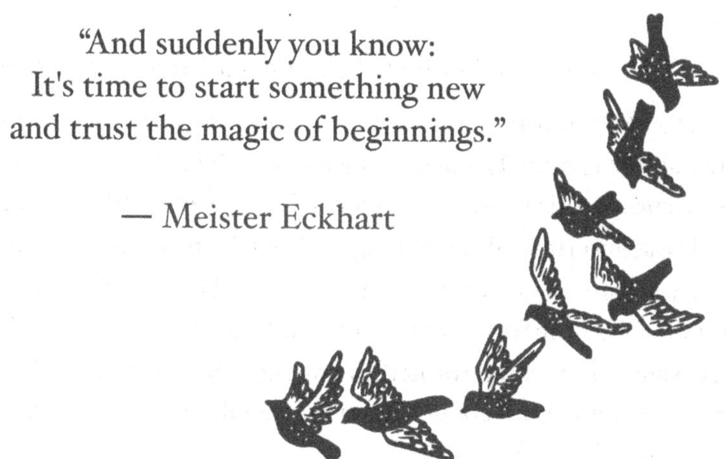

Flying Toward a New Dawn

It's almost my 24th birthday. I'm curled over my knees on the floor of a motel bathroom in western New York, crying in long, joyous release. I left California nine days ago in my truck, driving over all the grey, wintery landscapes of this country. It's December 9, 2001, and I'm on track to arrive to Massachusetts, and my old high school, by tomorrow. All kinds of men don't want me to say what I'm about to say. They've tried to stop me, called to "talk about content", sent letters, and now I'm done. I don't care what they want. I'm fucking thrilled to not care. Now I have a mini-speech prepared in my mind about my First Amendment rights, in addition to the longer speech I'm composing.

I've spoken my thoughts and my message into a mini-cassette recorder along the Interstates by day, then listened back and transcribed by night. I've slept under the camper shell in my Toyota pick-up each night of my journey so far. Now, I splurge on the motel room, so I can take a long shower and be refreshed when I get there. In the sweet clarity of the water, the ending of the speech comes to me. I step out. I'm warm, clean, and nestled into this steamy room, hurriedly writing down the final words in my notebook on the floor, '...because, there's infinite power and freedom in having nothing to hide'.

Then, after all I've been through, hearing my own voice and the power of these words releases the tears to flowing. When I crumple into crying there, it feels triumphant.

I know it will be ok. Better yet, it's going to be a whole new kind of ok; it's all going to be renewed in health. This is what I've been working towards for seven years. The darkness of their silencing and secrecy is about to end. I can feel a new day bursting forth from within me, like the light of truth refusing to be contained by darkness - in a body, in a school, or a society - any longer. It is coming. I'm happily floored by its power moving through me, literally bringing me to my knees.

The next day, my driving is calm, clear, and focused. Just four hours to go until I pull onto the familiar long driveway, up the rolling hills of this boarding school campus. The parking area is all quiet when I arrive, yet I know a great hum of energy is mounting inside. They know I'm coming, but do they know why? All three hundred-plus students, faculty and staff will be gathered in that auditorium. It's just me steering the Toyota with the California plates into a spot behind the back-stage entrance. I've decided I am not giving any one of them the chance to intercept me, no opening to pressure me to water down my message. I know these men. I know these tall, white colonial buildings. I can use that back door at ground level by the art studio and walk right onto stage-left.

It's bitter cold, as it always is in Massachusetts in December. My heart is thumping, but my sight is clear as I step out of the car. Mini-cassette recorder in hand. I inhale a chest-full of dry, cold New England air and see the steam of my breath as I step determinedly toward the doorway. It's unlocked, *Success!* I breathe in again, feeling the power and significance of what I am about to do. I pull the door open toward me and hear a full auditorium of young and old voices anxiously murmuring in anticipation. I step inside . . .

Roots

rad•i•cal răd'ĭ-kəl

adj. Arising from or going to a root or source; basic.
adj. Departing markedly from the usual or customary; extreme or drastic.
adj. Relating to or advocating fundamental or revolutionary changes in current practice, conditions or institutions.

Let's trace back to the roots, as the most radical place to begin, the way every being might enter this world with a longing to name the door through which they came. The urge is old, like the impossibly old, wise look on the face of a baby who seems to say without saying, '*I have seen so much.*'

We do this, trusting that we see as far back as our senses and memories will allow - yet, on other levels - we represent so much more than we can even grasp. We do not construct the framework of our entry-points, but the infinite possibility within is ours alone.

I was born just around the corner from Henry David Thoreau's Walden Pond, in Concord, Massachusetts, at the end of 1977. Later, I grew as a child in the town of Chelmsford, Massachusetts, bordering Jack Kerouac's

Lowell, with its old brick mills and the Merrimack River tracing a line of gritty history through all of my earliest memories.

My childhood was one of barefoot in trees, dirt on my hands and feet, horseback riding, nights spent awake watching shadows of leaves dance on the wall, and counting the grandfather clock tolls. So many siblings, breaking up fights, protecting the wounded, finding solace in silence - and always, the return to the safety of the trees.

There were grudgingly-attended country club outings, where adults held their breath while seeing and being seen among the fine table settings. I could sense they were saving true connection for another time, as was I in a way, with my ever-present longing to return to my rock walls and robin songs in the humid air. There were so many bike rides to the horse barn and, later, the sweet relief in writing.

I can still call up the sensations of those deciduous hardwood forests, with copper-colored floors of fallen leaves, the bitter smell of pines, moss on naked feet, and the eternal, mysterious stone walls from another time. I can smell the musty, green creek beds, alive with soil and water. We knew all the colors of seasons, lush green in summer with the sparkle of evening fireflies, dazzling golds, reds and orange in fall, and enduring white of serious winters.

I felt a connection to that landscape and its waters, even though the culture was discordant for me from the very beginning. If anything, the land became solace and respite from the culture. There was raucous energy and noise in the sheer size of my family (seven people in one house), balanced by immense stretches of timeless silence. The strangely stark contrast of the public and private. The ecstasy of the natural world and the hypocrisy of the societal. In all of these tensions, I grew.

Those New England village towns were ancient and eerie, stoic and charming. Us five kids could roam freely to "the center", a string of small businesses in modern 1980s shopping plazas and in 300-year-old colonials. The town was ours, and we fanned out into its old and newer corners with a wild crew of neighborhood kids among us. The five kids in my family, all born within six years (I was second, the oldest girl), represented the liveliest and most unruly force in town.

It was a fine place from which to set forth.

~ ~ ~

My parents came up in the poor and working class south, via Georgia, Tennessee, New Orleans and Florida. They met in junior college in Miami and married at 19 each, barely knowing themselves before seeking to recreate themselves in a new, northern region with a new socio-economic placement.

They took in a cultural story about money and status being a road to redemption. Their vision was of country clubs, fancy cars, expensive vacations, "fine things", and maybe an answer to a sense of worthiness that must have felt far out of reach. While I know now there is nothing to glorify in poverty, I also know my parents bought a lie and suffered in their own ways for it.

Like so many, they were rightly frustrated and disappointed when these things didn't satisfy or bring them any closer to one another. Their dissatisfaction was apparent to all of us kids from very early on, despite their efforts at a flawless, external image. They were what old-school New Englanders call "new money", reckless, excessive and short-sighted in their financial decisions. With a boundlessness of spending, they created an undercurrent of insecurity in our lives.

While nearly a million was spent on our high school educations, not a dime was saved for our college. The ironies were so many. The family home had a pool and a tennis court, yet our parents bought a condo with these same luxuries a three-hour drive away in New Hampshire. One year, they traveled to Europe, bought a Mercedes Benz from the manufacturer in Germany, and had it shipped across the ocean to Massachusetts (because, why buy local?). The car could travel the globe to reach them, but their goodwill could not travel over a kind word or the grace of true affection to reach each other.

So, we all stumbled slip-shod into the world of elitism, privilege among the wealthy, excess and debt, the luxury of the material while the internal and spiritual stifled and died.

Most importantly to this story, you must understand, my parents were perfectly primed to receive and not question a suggestion of being "not good enough" for the protections these elite institutions offered some. They had tried to answer the question of worthiness from the outside-in. This question remained unanswered for them as long as I lived at home, and seemed to continue unaddressed for many years afterward.

~ ~ ~

My grandparents came from Greece, Spain, England, Scotland, Ireland and the Native American plains.

While I was fortunate to have access to all four of them at some point in my life, my paternal Grandmother (of English, Scottish and Native American descent) was the brightest light in my family constellation's sky. For me, in addition to writing, silence, and the vast wisdom of the natural world, I most reveled in the gift of a clear-seeing Grandmother. Among these, she was my greatest salvation. She and I, too, lived in different worlds.

Esther "Connie" Fadjo loved the mall, the bright, bustling activity of Santa Monica, California, and all the new and stylish things. Her love for me was not conditional upon us meeting or relating in her world. She also marveled at mine. She would speak of the depths in my character and my love for the natural world with such a reverence. It was that of a person secure in themselves, who calmly and honestly sees another. Only through my Grandmother did I first come to understand the unique gifts that I bring.

Gramma was kind, sweet-natured and feisty-as-hell where it mattered. She could sing your praises with sincere and articulate flourish. Then, she could tell off the store clerk who tried to short-change her or make an inappropriate comment. She had worked, back in a time when women rarely did, writing the cryptic language of shorthand. She was wise and savvy with her resources. She was independent and also deeply loyal and loving. Her example of balancing these forces in one soul was a profound gift to me.

Us five kids felt the constant stress of our parents choices: too many children, too close together, and too much reckless consumerism. The tensions in their bond crackled inside a darkened chamber around us. That large house, then, was an echo chamber of pain most of the time. Then, every couple of years, Gramma and Grandpa would suddenly arrive. They were very much in love, and the whole resonance of the house changed when they entered it. They would stay for weeks or months at a time. Their presence was like the sun arriving, at last, to break up the clouds after a dark, tumultuous storm. Everything made sense when they were around. So, my childhood was punctuated with sunbursts of their presence.

The ultimate gift of my Grandmother was that we would sit in a light together, her welcoming me into the gaze of what is most important - knowing what is bullshit and what is true - and how to read the heart of a person. She taught me how to detect respect given or condescensions doled out. She saw the essence of what people brought to the world through how they lived, and her insights flung open many a door of understanding. She had incredibly beautiful hands. Our intermittent time together was a training for me. And a home for my heart.

~ ~ ~

Over the years, my parents exerted increasing pressure on me; to mold into a member of the society they most envisioned for themselves. Their vision soon clashed more and more with who I truly was. I began working at the horse barn at age ten, earning and saving my own money. I rode my bike four miles, there and back, up and down Robin Hill Road, and enjoyed a lot of independence for a girl my age. I recall my mother one day telling me to quit the horse barn and get a job at the dress shop in the center. It was even suggested once that I ride those horses side-saddle, instead of straddling them safely. I never did comply. I suppose I might have slid sideways off the beast of my wild nature and accepted a fate of docilely looking pretty in the center. In this way, I was always a disappointment.

I found more comfort in skateboarding with my three brothers, climbing trees late into childhood and doing yard work with my dad. Often, I was scolded for not being "lady-like" enough and pushed toward ideals that were absurd, disorienting and downright funny to me. I won't even talk about etiquette class in Boston. I got the message that I didn't understand what it meant to be a woman, and was eternally doing it wrong. Somehow, I was still waiting (unknowingly) for an example of womanhood beyond my Grandmother's, that I could actually embrace and identify with.

The chasms were wide. While there was love among individual family members, and joy in many moments, none of it was ever my place. I recall the distant sadness over this disconnect from early on, though it was always coupled with a fierce commitment to what I knew was true and good - in me and in the world. The sadness in childhood eventually yielded to a greater and greater fierceness as I came into myself.

This becomes relevant to the story, as well, because I was building a tolerance for the sensations of not belonging. You never know how your current pain will benefit you until much later. I began to rest in the knowing that it is always lonelier to be among people where you and your truth are not welcomed - than it ever is to be alone, owning and living your deepest truths.

I didn't know it at the time, but all of this would eventually serve me well.

The Stories We Tell - In the Beginning

Now, we pan back, with three stories for context: on faith, justice and shared values. First, Global concerned citizen Patrick Dodds shares in his stand-up act:

Let's talk about how we got here. As far as Western civilization is concerned, I think a lot of it comes back to the few major religions, all based on the same story. They are all founded on the story of Abraham. I'm sure you all know it. If you don't, I'll do a quick synopsis...

There's a guy named Abraham. God comes down and he says,

"Abraham, I want you to kill your son to please me."
Abraham replies, "God, do I gotta?"
"Yes, you gotta."
"I mean could I give you some gefilta fish or maybe a knish?"

"No, you must kill your son."

"Alright God, I'll do it.", Abraham replies. "Isaac! Isaac, come on boy. We're going on a good old father-son trip to the mountains. Just you and me, buddy. Just bring the knives and rope and we'll just have a good, old time."

God says, “Ha, no, Abraham, I was just messing with you. I was just pulling your leg. It’s alright. Just kill that poor, innocent, helpless animal instead and we’ll call it good.”

“Thanks God, that’s fine. You got it.”

And that’s how Western civilization essentially got started.

But!

What if a different Jewish person had been in that same situation. I am talking none other than Captain James T. Kirk. I’d be a different story, I tell you what...

“Captain Kirk, I want you to kill your son to please me.”

“Kill my son... Kill David. Oh, lord, but... No, I can’t do it. You get your bloodsport somewhere else, God. I couldn’t kill my son any more than you could kill yours.”

I put to you that humanity needs a better way. Not bloodshed but compassion.

“I beg you, don’t make me kill my son. You can send me to hell, but I won’t do it, mister. You hear me. I won’t do it.”

“Very good Captain, you have passed the test. You and your son and humanity may go in peace.”

Thank you, Patrick. Consider with me for a moment . . . *What if?*

~ ~ ~

Now, let's focus in on a certain time and place. In 1792, residents of Groton and Pepperell, Massachusetts, formed an association "for the purpose of erecting a suitable building, and supporting an Academy for superior educational purposes at Groton, Massachusetts."

This announcement was printed in the Columbian Centinel, a Boston newspaper of the time:

> *"This is to give notice, that a Public School is now opened in Groton, for the education of youth, of both sexes" in which School are taught the English, Latin and Greek Languages, Writing, Arithmetic, Geography, the Art of Speaking and Writing, with Practical Geometry, and Logic".*

Yet, this School faced financial hardship 76 years later, when "an errant firecracker" on the Fourth of July 1868 set fire to the buildings. Despite the original, published intention of "education of youth, of both sexes", they sought self-preservation at the expense of young women. They denied women entry for seventy-three years. As if by some act of god (as it is often called), the school endured yet another major fire in 1956. This time at a graduation ceremony, during this boys-only period.

Their motto in Latin is "Omnibus Lucet", meaning, "Let Light Shine Upon All". *Does it?*

~ ~ ~

In the same year, 1792, George Washington was re-elected president, preparing to serve in the second-ever term of that office. The ideals and practices of a democratic government were still young and experimental. Settlers from Europe on a foreign continent had declared their Independence from Britain, a mere sixteen years earlier, stating:

In every stage of these Oppressions We have Petitioned for Redress in the most humble terms: Our repeated Petitions have been answered only by repeated injury. A Prince whose character is thus marked by every act which may define a Tyrant, is unfit to be the ruler of a free people.

Meanwhile, the first Columbus Day Celebration was held in 1792 in New York City, 300 years after his arrival in North America. This explorer and colonizer had a dark history of tyranny and brutality. A Spanish historian named Consuelo Varela says, "Even those who loved him had to admit the atrocities that had taken place." Meanwhile, native people in what we know as Ohio and the Great Lakes Region were actively fighting The United States Army in the "Ohio" or "Little Turtles War". This government-sanctioned violence against indigenous people destroyed many, many lives.

In these simultaneous accounts, within the story of a newly forming people, it becomes unclear. Was brutality among men condemned or celebrated?

On Education

"Education is simply the soul of a society
as it passes from one generation to another."

— Gilbert K. Chesterton

In 1986, my parents shifted all five of us kids from education at the local Chelmsford, Massachusetts public schools to the private Notre Dame Academy, a parochial Catholic school just south of the New Hampshire border in Tynsgboro, Massachusetts. I entered in the third grade to a class of about 48 students, eight of which were boys. The school had only recently gone "co-ed". Women in habits walked somberly down cavernous halls with too-tall ceilings, sisters of a holy order, nuns, and lay teachers. It was a massive institution, backed by an indomitable Church with a much longer history.

You could say that Catholicism was atmospheric in my childhood. Irish-Catholics, Italian-Catholics (along with other ethnicities I couldn't name) were the companions at most of our civic events and outings. Though, my best childhood friend was Jewish, and I learned to wear the kippah or yarmukle head covering and light the candles on Friday evenings in their home. Chelmsford, Massachusetts, had a Catholic church right across the street from my father's dental office. We kids weren't required to go to mass with our father on Sundays. Though, if we did brave the journey at 6 am, he would treat us to Burger King french toast sticks afterward.

I appreciated that participation in "religion" was optional at home. Yet, it was required at Notre Dame Academy. The more I saw at school, the more I longed for something I missed or something I hadn't known yet.

The 'ruler on the knuckles' thing was passé by the 1980s, but I did watch a nun grab a boy by the collar and throw him up against the wall in front of the whole line of us children. I watched another nun throw a different student's papers out the third-story window in some fit of unexplained rage. Worst was a memory of one particularly disturbing nun coming into class one day and simply facing the blackboard, with her back to us. It was a morning like any other, and it took some time for the class to quiet down and notice the oddity of her behavior. Once we were sufficiently unnerved and silenced, she was satisfied enough to speak.

Still facing the wall and not her silent, motionless students, she bellowed, "You know, there is no justice in this world." We all felt nervous. She continued, "My father died last night, and you kids can't even do your homework!". What the hell are 10-year-old kids supposed to do with that? She vented and huffed a while longer, and then we proceeded to the business of the day. Some icky sense of exaggerated guilt and confusion lingered about us and became a constant cloud of stifled emotions. It became the polluted air we breathed at Notre Dame Academy of Tyngsboro, Massachusetts.

Of course, beauty can exist in the darkest of places. There was one very kind nun who extended a generosity toward me during my fifth-grade year. One day, as I approached her desk by her beckon, she said in hushed tones, "Vanessa, you march to the beat of a different drummer." At eleven years old, I truly had no idea what she meant, or whether or not this was a good thing.

I worried that I was again getting in trouble, but in some way I couldn't understand. Then, her countenance softened some, and I slowly began to relax, too. She said, "You hold on to that. It might not be the easiest life, but it will bring you great things."

Sister (I truly cannot recall her name) gave me my own wall at the Art Fair - art being the absolute highlight of my days at NDA. She offered her quiet support to me, almost under the radar. I offer up my gratitude for that.

> "If a man does not keep pace with his companions,
> perhaps it is because he hears a different drummer.
> Let him step to the music which he hears,
> however measured or far away."
>
> — Henry David Thoreau

I recognize now, there has been a constant stream of people in my life who have celebrated and encouraged me along, even from within corrupt structures. It was as if they saw a spirit in me they admired, yet had to do so quietly, lest they threaten their chosen position within the system. I imagine each one lived a contrast of inner hopes and outer realities, recognizing some possibility of a life unfolding where things could be different.

I could hear their voices, *"Look, I can't go there because I'm too dug-in. But you could! Go, sweet and brave soul. I celebrate every one of your successes from the inside."* That "there" is any form of liberation which requires a touch of defiance, a commitment to your own truth, and a fierceness to sustain you as you meet resistance. I wonder as I grow more fully into adulthood, about the concessions people will make, and the tradeoffs. What is the cost of securing our place in what-already-is, and what are the benefits? How can we fulfill our destinies inside an upside-down value system, without sacrificing the best of who we are?

I left NDA at the end of eighth grade in 1992, after 'doing six years', as I like to put it. Hell, even the buildings were shaped like penitentiaries. I kept one good friend and a wry sense of rebellious humor at any excess of imprisonment and control. I earned my Get Out of Jail Free Card - and would soon find the greater freedoms and complexities that lay beyond.

~ ~ ~

I arrived as a student at Lawrence Academy of Groton, Massachusetts in the fall of 1992, the year of their bicentennial celebration. My older brother, Damon, was already there, two grades ahead of me. My sister, Adrienne, would arrive the following year, one grade behind me.

These boarding schools are like mini-college campuses, with sprawling, manicured lawns of green cradling stately buildings of brick and white. It's a little overdone for young people ages 13-19, to be honest. This superimposing of two life stages evokes a feeling like watching toddlers try on their parents' work shirt: optimism and a touch of tender humor. The prestigious image reassures parents that their kids will be going onto real universities, by the facade of similarity. This marketing approach echoes the embarrassingly overblown prom ritual, in the gesture to say, '*Yes, like that*'. Elite boarding high schools are to ivy-league universities what the prom ritual is to the institution of marriage. Somehow, kids and adults willingly participate in it all as a 'real-life' dress-rehearsal.

I recall the exaggerated hype leading up to my first days on campus, as a 13-year-old. There was nervous expectation around entrance exams and the browsing of glossy, boarding school catalogs in advance. I always felt like I was on someone else's ride. This world and all it seemed to represent was a foreign land, and I was an eternal stranger in it. Or, maybe the apparent positional distance was intentional. They wanted you to know they were *Big*, and you now had to step up.

Becoming a Lawrence Academy student had its own pressures, all of which were placed on us young people and not the adults. We were expected to prove ourselves worthy. I also recall the school not being our first choice - neither mine nor our family's. Still, it was the first stop on the train to "the outside" after parochial school, so I rode with relief all the same. I just don't think I was ever the one to choose the destination. It certainly wasn't my map anyone referenced.

Still, I savored every one of the new freedoms: my own clothes, a balanced mix of genders to live among, art classes, the ability and encouragement to be active in my body. I soon fell in love with modern dance. I made connections with people I could respect completely because they were forming identities on who they were - not what a strict God-fearing system said they could and could not be. If I did not relate to the destination, I definitely came to love the other travelers.

Dethroning - the Seat of Authority

That first year is a bit of a blur for me, though I did meet groundskeeper, Peter Regis, toward the end of the year. I'd been a 'tomboy' of the 1980s, spending hours of my childhood working alongside my dad in the yard. So there was a familiarity in our dynamic for me. I don't remember how the meeting happened, or what he used as a means to approach my friends and me. But, I was familiar with an older man taking me under his wing to show me traditionally male-oriented skills. I longed for those skills to become a more balanced and capable human being. Soon, he was teaching me about cars in his shop.

Peter Regis was a ragged-looking man of about 40 then, though, to me, he seemed to be much further into middle age. That's the thing about perspective and youth. It will all look a certain way from a certain place. For the young, that means things look bigger than they truly are. Predators know this. Pete led an Automotive workshop for students every March when kids engaged in experiential learning. So, he regularly hosted kids in his shop. I had every reason to trust that he was a good and honorable man. He was more than a maintenance person on campus; he was a teacher of sorts. He and his wife lived among students in the boys' dormitory called Waters.

By my second year, I wanted to expand my newfound freedom to living on campus. My relationship with my mom had always been tense and painful. My parents were unhappy. I was craving as much independence in the world as possible, as quickly as I could get it. I was granted this wish. So, at the beginning of my sophomore year, I moved onto campus and into the Dr. Green dormitory.

~ ~ ~

That year, when a group of friends and I were caught for smoking, we stood in headmaster Steve Hahn's opulent, cathedral-like office while he floundered through some response. This man was absurdly tall, with a tuft of curly brown hair over thinly rimmed-glasses, and a seemingly constant little grin that didn't fit any situation. It was as if his head were contentedly in the clouds, just high enough to not concern himself with the real happenings of those below him. It was hard to tell what place he spoke from when he did. Did he actually see us or register where he was? What was he even saying? I recall that nothing of his way of being inspired trust.

As about six of us students stood in a ring, he tried to speak of his position and how difficult it was for him. He said, "Would any of you like to be in my position?". I raised my hand. Since he had set the stage, even unwittingly, we followed through on the enactment. I sat in the big chair in his grand office and acknowledged the efforts the kids were making to keep the area clean. I expressed my concerns for their health and started outlining ways they could become better citizens... until it all ended in an eruption of teenage giggles.

Now I see the significance of that moment: his offering the chair. For in a way, the choices he was about to make would become a dethroning of sorts. The chair of authority sat empty. Nobody was claiming the spot in which to say, "This is the right thing to do. This is how a leader of a school responds and serves its families. Here is what must be done". Those words would not be spoken from that chair. So, I would soon be compelled to assume the post for a full seven years.

~ ~ ~

Amidst great joy and freedom with my friends, another layer of life in the new place began to reveal itself to me. The darkness beneath the projection screen of prestige was spreading outward, touching the lives of more and more people in proximity. While I savored freedoms and love among classmates, a stark contrast suddenly emerged.

Confusing things started to happen. Exchanges with Pete that left me feeling uncertain and unsettled. It was a progression of subtle, intentional confusions of the line between mentor, friend, caregiver, and adult man in authority. If a bunch of us kids were living there on campus, and these adults were our daily caretakers, what was the appropriate line?

There were times, he'd pretend to be out of sight, but be closer than you'd expect. There was the time he pretended he was in pain and needing help. All trickery. Every one was part of a formula this man had crafted over (I would soon learn) decades to create unhealthy, unsafe situations. Misleading and abusing kids.

I ache to know that so many people reading now know exactly what I'm talking about. Abuse of power thrives on intentional confusion. This will appear repeatedly, later, and throughout this story. Just pay special attention, here, to the fact that moving a line of acceptable around and framing moments one way, while acting as if they are another, is the territory of abuse.

The urge to trust is so strong. The drive to believe that we have been right in trusting is also a crucial aspect of maintaining our health. As social creatures, we thrive in connection. Young people especially need to believe that those they have trusted are, in fact, worthy of that trust. We all depend on those older than us to help us survive in the world while we grow.

How could it be anything different?

Luckily for me, Pete slipped a comment one day that helped to bring this contrast, and a new awareness, very clearly into focus for me. After he'd pretended, and blurred lines, and deceived, he finally said, "It may be best to not say anything to anyone, in case they get the wrong idea.".

Ah, ha. The moment of contrasting realities was finally right there before me. In an instant, my sight on the world expanded. Painful and ugly, but at least perfectly clear. We may not like what we see when our sight expands. But, at least we can work with clear.

Keep something a secret for you?

Hell No, my friend. I don't care who you are.

~ ~ ~

I quickly told the people closest to me: my boyfriend, Blake, and my closest friends. After someone in a position of authority abuses their power, you naturally feel less inclined to trust other adults in the same setting. Those kinds of violations of trust call into question everything you think you know about grown-ups, schools, and the right order of the world. If this was a place that had people like that, it never once occurred to me to tell any other faculty or staff member.

Even as an adult, I think that is a valid question. How far would tolerance for that kind of behavior reach in the place?

I sure as F didn't ever think of telling headmaster, Steve Hahn.

Within weeks, a close friend approached me to say Pete Regis was doing similar things to her. By now, it was spring, and events started unfolding very quickly. While I didn't tell any adult, this point bears repeating: It's crucially important to tell someone. Preferably, a few someones. Because she knew what I'd been through, my friend felt safe to come to me with that information. Of course, it was relevant because I'd seen similar behavior in Pete, and because I cared for her very much. There is always someone who will understand and care very much. Always.

Now, Blake, Sybil, and I could see a pattern. We had each other, and we had a fierce love for one another.

It was time for action.

Major Blessing - Friendship

"Friendship is a sheltering tree."

— Samuel Taylor Coleridge

"Every oak tree started out
as a couple of nuts who stood their ground."

— Henry David Thoreau

Sybil came in as a freshman during my sophomore year, and we were on the same soccer team. She's the kind of person who carries a tough exterior yet is all big heart and kindness beneath. She seemed shy, with her head down, and also full of intelligence and depth. You know those kinds of people hold magnitudes inside if they'd only become willing to grace the world with their depths. I liked her right away.

We first connected deeply on a bus trip to an 'away' game. Her steady, quiet way was endearing to me, and our conversations were soothing, warm, and even giddy. We eventually shared campouts on her parents 100 acres in Central Massachusetts, went to numerous Ani DiFranco concerts, and spent many a languid hour in deep conversation. Different as we were, there was a tender, intuitive understanding between us, which continued for so many years to come.

Then, that spring of 1994, we suddenly had a shared mission. Once she and I started talking about Pete Regis, there were soon rumblings among other acquaintances about their encountering similar things. It was bigger than one or two confusing moments with an authority figure who overstepped and overstepped. It was a phenomenon.

Soon enough, we knew, the way kids always know what's really going on, that this man had managed to reach the highest levels of sexual offense with a few students. We had these stories among us now, and the urgency of our task grew. We understood then, as we do now, that the choice to reveal that kind of experience belongs solely to the individual. We could honor that, even as we were awed by the enormity of what this all meant. It was the most pressing thing occupying our days.

So, we skipped soccer practice and met under a tree one afternoon. We started by writing out our feelings and thoughts on what was happening. Then, we took turns sharing. It was powerful to name it all, to have words deliver that pain out of our bodies where we could both hear it spoken. The added sense of sound confirmed the inner reality. It was cathartic, releasing that agony, and then, just being quiet and accepting with one another.

Mine was written as if I was speaking to Pete. "You have no right to act that way. It is wrong what you are doing". I went last, and those words, with all of their power, lingered in the air between us. It arose spontaneously then, what needed to happen next. We would go down there together, and I would read that to him, what I had written.

Holy shit, that was potent for a 16-year old.

I told Blake what we planned to do, and he said he would skip baseball practice and wait outside with his bat. I remember him respectfully bringing up what I would wear for the confrontation. In his protective male wisdom, he suggested I choose something that played down my body and sexuality. I remember I wore a navy blue long dress with a wrap-around sweater. It's funny what you remember. He may have wanted to go in there and take action himself, but he had strength enough to balance his urges with giving us our moment. He would be just outside the door, he told us, listening.

The day arrived. Sybil and I met up, full of jitters, and began the walk down to the garage in silence. We locked eyes and nodded, our gaze speaking everything we needed to say and unifying us into sharp focus. We were doing this.

When we entered the shop together, full of presence and determination, Pete seemed to know right away what was happening. We stood in opposition, he and us. My hands were shaking horribly as I began. I spoke, "What you are doing is wrong. You have no right to act that way", and on it flowed. The steady faith of my friend fed me with strength, and I let it pour out from me. I was speaking for me, for her, for all of our friends, for something even beyond that.

Luckily, Pete hung his head and nodded and agreed with everything we said.

Sybil, Blake, and I reunited in a thrill of relief and exhilaration outside. We ran up away from those doors, breathing heavily and laughing a bit from the sheer power of it. We spontaneously decided to take that piece of paper and burn it. We wanted to see it all washed away. To see it disintegrate into the air - the disease, dysfunction, and attempted theft of that which was not his - just evaporating into the sky. We huddled together and let the fire and smoke work its magic. Speaking for myself, I truly believed that would mark the end of it.

There was massive relief for each of us, and a good buzz among our friend group about what had happened. Soon after, a grown woman who worked in the local pizza shop downtown found me to quietly say thank you. She told me, Pete had done the same things to her when she was our age.

That meant this man had been deceiving and preying on girls for at least a decade. Holy shit, indeed.

~ ~ ~

A friend of ours, also on the soccer team, soon decided to tell a teacher. I pieced this all together in reverse from stories shared later on. That was the right thing to do. She hadn't been rattled by these experiences and could more clearly decide who would and would not be a trustworthy adult here. In my memory, I know which friend relayed the information and which teacher passed it on to administration. Their taking action sent a message, "This is important. Something needs to be done about this.". I won't say those names here. But please know, if you are reading and you recognize yourself (friend or teacher)... Thank you.

Friendship was the blessing that galvanized me into action. That confrontation was borne of love for a friend and an urge for protection of many others. I may not have known yet how to look out for and protect myself - but I knew how to protect those I loved.

I honestly don't know how it would have worked otherwise. When someone in a power position abuses the dynamic, the isolation for the vulnerable person is enough to create a confusion that can linger for years. I tip my hat to those who've found the conviction and clarity in themselves to declare that their private experience mattered enough for a reckoning. Some people call this the heart of integrity. Regardless of what gender, race, sexual orientation, or class you currently identify with, I know every one of you can appreciate the courage of that journey - from deep inner knowing to outward confrontation.

You might be thinking of a situation or a relationship that could use some rebalancing right now...

Remember, it is always worth the risk to open your heart and the honesty of your pain to someone you trust, even when what you hold there seems awful and scary. Even if you fear it could disqualify you from love. So often, the opposite is true.

Sybil would become my right-hand-gal in so many things, with so many firsts and shared adventures together. We were about to face yet another.

The Door Through Which You Came, The First Door

Just days after our confrontation with Pete, Sybil and I got matching hand-written notes in our school mailboxes. "Please come to my office at 2 pm on May 18. - Steve Hahn". We didn't know what to expect, but we went in together all the same. When we entered, a whole circle of adults sat with serious, expectant faces, and told us to have a seat. With scarcely an introduction, we were then ordered to answer questions and give details to these authority figures and a stranger.

Where we had celebrated our accomplishment with Pete, this was no party. There was no acknowledgment of what we'd gone through, nor any gratitude for what we'd done to stop this terrible thing. A true disagreement was surfacing: we believed it was obviously wrong for this man to be molesting girls on campus and needed to be stopped - they believed this was not a big deal, something to keep quiet and tolerate.

Of course, they were simply covering their legal asses. The meeting, therefore, was in service to them, and the intentions showed.

In Sybil's words many years later, "We were heard in that we were expected to tell our experiences. And though the experience was not quite hostile, I don't recall feeling very supported by the leaders of our school to protect my friend, to protect other girls, to protect me."

That we were so outnumbered, that our parents were not involved in this meeting - most of all - that we were excused with absolutely no information about what would happen next. All of it was the early revelation of their true motivations in this situation.

We were just 14 and 16, respectively. But, we knew in our hearts the significance of this. We knew that so many had been affected by this man's actions. Every adult in that room failed to register the importance or show any humane response to the obvious atrocity. We met only blank faces and shut down hearts. We knew it was all wrong.

Worst of all, we heard nothing more from any faculty or staff on campus about it. Not a word. I returned to my classes and to my dorm each night, the mystery of what-came-next closing in around me. Then, a few days later, I woke early - maybe 6 am in the dim light - to a rumbling noise outside my window. Pete Regis was out there, circling the front lawn of Dr. Green on his tractor and looking up at my window. Thank all things good that I lived on the second floor. My heart was racing, and I felt remarkably alone. What could I do, and who could I tell?

The highest-up people in the school knew all about it. I'd found the courage to walk into his shop with Sybil and tell him he was wrong. But, there he was still. He could roam freely, and his presence felt menacing, volatile. What was he there to do?! I felt trapped. My dorm mother was an especially obnoxious younger woman, who always exuded an air of condescension toward us kids. I'd pieced together earlier that year, that she had overheard details about my personal life as I talked to my roommate and passed them on to other students. She would be no help.

I felt frozen and with nowhere to go for protection. In my panic, I believed I could only wait. I carefully watched and managed my alarm, until Pete drove away on his tractor.

I went into Steve Hahn's office that day and said I needed to talk. Perhaps there was just a delay between this discovery and the action or consequence. I asked, "What is going to happen now, with Pete?". Steve Hahn said smugly, "Pete has been placed on a kind of suspension contract [a term used for student discipline]. If he has contact with students again, he has to leave". I was stunned. None of that made sense. He scooted me out of there, with a look of terror on my face as I attempted to digest what he was saying to me. He was saying they were going to do nothing.

As you can imagine, I had a hell of a time trying to fall asleep in my dorm after that. Pete was a groundskeeper; he did maintenance on all of the buildings. Did he have a key to the dorm? To say I became hyper-vigilant would be an understatement. I did not have my friend beside me. My boyfriend lived in the dorm further down the quad. He wouldn't hear me if I needed help.

A few days later, Pete came again and stood unselfconsciously on the lawn, staring up at my window. Somehow, without the tractor, his presence was more unsettling. He wasn't even pretending to be casually doing something else. By now, he was standing there blankly, defiantly watching me. I was fucking terrified. I hid and prayed and got the blessing of one more safe start to a day, as he wandered off on foot.

I went to Steve Hahn again. I said, "Look, we have to do something about this. It's not ok that Pete is still on campus. I don't feel safe." I don't remember his words exactly. But, his response was so intentionally unclear that the intentions soon became very clear. He was bullshitting me. I essentially said, *'Um, your response to this is entirely inadequate.'* I was pointing out the obvious. Maybe it was the first time someone challenged his behavior, and truly, he had no worthy response.

'Oh, yes, we'll look into it, and see what we can do', he offered, as words with no substance or integrity. He hollowed himself out with false promises. I did my best to resume my 16-year-old life of classes, sports, and sleeping in that dorm. Yet, I heard nothing still. At least, I didn't hear what I expected.

~ ~ ~

The year was wrapping up quickly. It was nearly graduation, and prom was happening somewhere amidst all this. There was always a flurry of activity as the year ended. But one day, Steve Hahn called me into his office again. I stood there alone. He stood as well. There was one other adult as a silent witness. I remember this person sat in a chair.

Steve then informed me, "There is no financial aid available for you to come back next year." My head started spinning. It wasn't just the words; there was something dark and cold in what he was communicating to me. I desperately wanted to make sense of it, but that urge kept meeting dissonance as the reality came to me again and again.

He continued, "We only had enough money for one of the Fadjo's to come back, so your sister will be attending next year." What?! Then, I remember the oddest sensation. I felt like my soul, my best self, started to float away. I became dizzy. The visual of that tall, ridiculous man stood before me, and the ominous blank-faced character in the chair receded into a fog, too. I was floating away as the blood rushed to my major organs, and I was lightheaded. This was really happening. I was being punished and sent away. I would not be allowed to come back next year.

My heart probably leapt to all of my friends, my first love. I could feel all of it being taken away from me. I knew so plainly I wasn't in the wrong, and yet here they were, making me the one to pay. I couldn't process all of that in a moment. In truth, it would take years. I recall a phrase was sometimes thrown around, about a kid being "not invited back". Was that said by Steve Hahn then? Or did I hear it in my own ears, as some puzzle-piecing together of the terrible ways this school leveraged its power? Here, where 'private', meant, 'therefore, able to do whatever the hell we want'. I didn't know. I knew something terrible was happening to me.

I could barely stand up straight.

~ ~ ~

The world was suddenly and utterly changed. The place where I stood was abruptly torn from its roots, right there beneath my feet, severing the connection between what was right and what was wrong. We were all drifting there in a netherland of impossibility, in a fog of their own creation. For years, I would later have dreams of a house being picked up off its foundation and spun in the air, just like Dorothy and Toto in the Wizard of Oz. It was always an echo of that moment.

You can walk through some doors many times, and it is always the same door.

There are some doors, though, you can only walk through so many times. Then, things change. Sometimes, you will walk through that old door until you are no longer the same person who walked through it before. Your sight becomes wider, and your ability to see and feel the truth of what lies on each side, far broader. In that way, you walk through a door for the very first time. Same doorway, different threshold.

That spring, I walked through the doors of the headmaster's office as a trusting student, willing to accept their authority and their story, for the very last time.

I was acutely and painfully aware now, they had chosen where to let their loyalties lie. They were not with me, a child whose family had given so much for me to be there. They were not behind me, not with my courage in speaking up to protect other students. The school's loyalties were with the child molester.

The world, and my place in it, would never be the same.

Nearly Ran Away

Figuring out what came next, after being sent away, was stumbling and awful all the way through. Plans were set initially for me to attend Westford Academy for my junior year, the smaller public high school bordering my home town of Chelmsford, Massachusetts. I felt fine enough about this next course of action, given that I was now safer, relatively, and away from the stalking child molester. My soul was starting to shut down, and this is a feeling to which I will always be highly attuned. You must catch it before it catches you. It is a slippery slope that runs a very real risk of swallowing the best of us whole. It can happen while we're feeling numb, too, so the awareness is especially important.

By that first summer, I was only starting to calm myself. I knew I would have to adjust to living with the grief of losing daily contact with my friends and with Blake. With so much lost, all I could do was begin to get new bearings on my life.

Then, my parents informed me - just weeks before the start of school - that I would instead go to Bishop Guertin, the parochial co-ed high school just over the border in New Hampshire. My brother Cameron would be attending. Maybe they figured, with me at 16, and able to drive, this would make life easier. I could drive both of us to school. But, and I choose this word very intentionally, the place was hell.

The contrast to life on "the outside" I'd thrived in for two years was screaming at me as I entered the penitentiary scene again. I'd released those particular shackles, and their weight was even heavier this time around, knowing what I knew. I saw some of the same kids who'd gone to my elementary school. The adjoining Notre Dame Academy High School was still girls-only, so Bishop Guertin captured all the boys whose parents wanted parochial high school for their sons. I did not want a revisit.

I'd spoken up to the injustice and obvious wrong of Steve Hahn knowingly employing a child molester and was sent away. Now, adults in my world were asking me to walk back into confinement. I was frustratingly stuck in that stage of growth where you are subject to your parents' dictates, yet wise enough to legitimately challenge it all. I rattled inside a terrible dissonance on the edge of emancipation.

I suppose it was the part of me that still had a tolerance for my soul shutting down. Maybe the sadness had taken over. But, either way, come September, I put on my uniform and drove Cameron and myself up to New Hampshire to Bishop Guertin High School.

On day two, the teacher had all of us stand at the side of a desk, while they inspected every adolescent to ensure that our uniforms were up to standard. Being terrified of human sexuality as they were, there was always a focus on the sufficient length of the girl's skirt. The socks had to be knee-high (apparently, knees can be the only un-sexy part of the exposed female body), and all details buttoned up. We stood stiff and still as the teacher slowly paced the aisles, inspecting. Think, Tim Robbins in Shawshank Redemption.

Then, on day four, I'd forgotten my lunch in my car. I told someone I needed to go out and get it. They instructed me to wait at the door, while another faculty member was sent for, to escort me to my car and back. What? I was not even allowed the freedom to walk to my car alone to get a sack lunch, or trusted to return obediently. I snapped.

The next day, I woke in a daze and slowly put on my uniform in a fog. Then, I started crying in the bathroom. I could not stop crying. Something essential to my soul's health was being taken away, and I was suffocating under the restraint of this system. The tears were a good sign - they meant I had not died inside - and that which sought freedom was bucking against the circumstances. I was amazed at all the uncontrollable crying. Eventually, the tears stopped, and I had peace. By the time I left the house with my younger brother, I had become resolute. Something had shifted, and I'd decided the inner life of my soul would win.

I drove up to that big, stoic building in New Hampshire and pulled the car over to the curb. Cameron looked at me and asked, "What are you doing?". I said firmly, "I'm not going." He was stunned, laughed a little nervously. But, he was not surprised. I said, "I don't know where I'm going, but you'll have to get a ride home with someone else. Can you ask your friend for a ride?". Clearly registering my unwavering stance on this, Cameron nodded with a concerned look on his face and got out of the car. "Good." I said.

Then, I fucking drove.

I just kept driving. I was raging, and miserable, and the insanity of all I was being buffeted about by - standing up to Pete Regis, losing my place and my friends, the absolute absurdity of schools like Bishop Guertin even existing - it was cascading around me in overpowering waves. I could not succumb to it. There was too much of my very life force at stake. I needed a way out, with my truest self intact.

I was pointed west, as that was where Blake and I had talked about going after high school. We dreamed of traveling to California together, and I was drawn to all that land west of all I'd known. I wasn't exactly thinking straight at the moment. I was just going now. I'd made it to the New York state border when the practical details started to come back to me. I wasn't prepared. I was wearing that ridiculous uniform and I had no supplies. I would at least need to go back and gather my crucial things - or stop at a thrift shop and build up from scratch. Could I return and escape again, under the cover of night? Where was I going?

Still focused, but no longer raging, I drove to the home of a friend in Central Massachusetts to clear my head. I needed to talk through my plan with someone who cared about me, and her place was first on Route 2 East, back toward supplies. I'd spent the day driving, and she was home now from school - her parents just cleaning up after dinner. We went up into her room. I said I had to go, and she understood. In our young and imagination-filled way, we talked over what I could do.

My friend's parents slowly became aware of the intensity of the situation and my plans. They saw a young woman who was simply in a tight place, and needed to find a way through. Her father was the one to approach us, and his calm, wise alliance reached me as respect. He didn't try to talk me out of running away. He just spoke to the part of me that was in pain. He said, "Look, when you talk to your parents about this, I would take the, 'I'm really unhappy' position, and leave the running away part for another time."

As a parent now, I can imagine the precarious responsibility they must have felt in that moment. You know your child's friend is going to run away at 16 - and you have the potential power to guide her toward some kind of safety. I stayed into the evening and eventually made my way back to my parent's house. The first version of my plan was cut short, but my determination remained. I imagine all the hours my parents spent wondering where I was, combined with Cameron's story, brought enough gravity to the situation that they simply yielded.

I do not remember what came next, but I never put on that uniform again.

~ ~ ~

By some process of compromise or brain-storming, I registered as a junior at Acton-Boxboro Regional High School. Acton, Massachusetts borders the town of Concord, where I was born, and made for a mere 20-minute drive down Route 27 from Chelmsford. I was late in starting, but with this vast sea of young people, no one seemed to care or notice. Now, this may have been, and may be now, a fine example of public schooling at its best. I don't actually know. My time at Acton-Boxboro was marked only by anonymity and a sense of being untracked and untraceable. 'No one cares' was the general sentiment under which I survived. They didn't care, and neither did I.

I remember having an advisor, actually called "Mr. Clever", who told me in exasperation one day late in the year, "Vanessa, Acton-Boxboro is the real world, and you're going to have to get used to it.". There was the voice of misplaced authority, again. Here was another man, trying to define the whole world for a woman for whom nothing was truly working. Whatever defeat he was trying to transfer on to me, I did not accept. No matter how clever he might believe himself to be.

This was a school of 3,000 kids, where Lawrence Academy had been one of 300. I floated along, taking in the first glimpses of a vast, mainstream way of doing high school. I was there often enough. But, I was only biding my time. I had chosen not to risk running away that day, so I bargained out the consequences and figured I'd have some fun doing it. I soon took my life savings of $800 and bought myself my very first car. Freedom was approaching in incremental steps. I took a job at the new pizzeria in Chelmsford and started saving money again that way.

I barely went to school. I believe I had the second-highest "tardies" ranking in the school. The true honor went to a buddy of mine named Adam. I used to pick him up at his home in Acton on my way in sometimes. He had big eyes and a wide, kind face. I quickly found my people at Acton-Boxboro, the artsy-natural-free-spirited folks who made my time there livable. Skipping school was not only easy, it became a way of life for me. Given all I'd seen, why would I give any adult or institution my respect? I was biding my time until the age of emancipation - 18 - arrived, and it was merely a game to me.

As soon as I was legally able to do it, I would run away for good.

Useful Skills - Not Caring What People Think

"Great spirits have always encountered violent opposition from mediocre minds."

— Albert Einstein

"The one thing that doesn't abide by majority rule is a person's conscience."

— Harper Lee

I recall a weekend at home in Chelmsford the year before, when my grandparents were fortunately in town. I was annoyed and sulking over being caught and reprimanded for smoking cigarettes on the Lawrence Academy campus. Whatever faculty member found me made sure to lay down all the accompanying burdens of guilt and shame. Gramma said, "Oh, to hell with them, Nessa. I smoked and drank and danced, and I turned out just fine.".

Gramma had mastery over this crucial skill: Not Caring What People Think.

It wasn't easily won, of course, as is so often the case. Her father had been a Baptist preacher in the farmlands of southern California in the 1920s & 30s when she came of age. He had admonished her constantly for all the 'sins' she'd enjoyed, forever trying to steer her away from damnation. She cultivated this skill by growing a resistance to his harshness and criticisms and still choosing to be herself anyway.

I'd had some early "not caring what people think" training, by being just as tomboyish or un-ladylike as had suited me in childhood. Now, in my teens, I had extra practice as my identity was becoming more and more my own. Gramma's perspective, reveling in the freedom on the other side of those criticisms, was so helpful.

My youngest brother once told me, when I was about 17 and he 14, that what he admired in me most was that I didn't care what people think. That same year, I had picked him up from school one day at Notre Dame Academy, where he was still a student. My brother, Travis, was a skateboarder and into the punk scene. He experimented with shaving his head on both sides and using the ironing board to flatten spikes of hair straight up into a 'mohawk'.

So, on this afternoon, a nun escorted my younger brother all the way to the car after school. She stood there grumbling some discouraging, shaming language about him as he climbed into the front seat. Like I'd let that go unaddressed. As she turned to walk away, I rolled that window down and bellowed, "You know, Travis, you shouldn't have to go to school where people treat you like *shit!*".

Perhaps Not Caring What People Think arises when you decide you care even more about something truly meaningful to you. I loved my little brother, and no one was going to talk about him that way under my watch. I still consider his, "The thing I admire about you most..." comment to be his highest compliment to me.

It is a paradox and a blessing - that in caring deeply, and committing to the right and true, we are freed from caring about other things.

Let's consider the classic social experiment by Solomon Asch, from 1951. Subjects were introduced to a test (of line lengths) where there was an obvious wrong answer. Sure, for the sake of experimental thought, let's keep in mind that obvious wrong answer I'd witnessed in 1994 at Lawrence Academy. In this experiment, a "naive" participant is introduced to a group of seven (actually-called) "stooges".

The stooges agree in advance what the correct answer will be. All the while, the naive participant believes everyone is on equal footing in the situation (glossy catalog, perhaps?). Then, each participant - all male in this case - states aloud their answer to, 'Which two lines are the same size?'. Again, the answer is designed to be obvious. The naive participant, having entered most recently, would give his answer last.

Asch found that about 1/3 (32%) of participants always went along with the clearly-wrong majority answer. Over the 12 critical trials, about 75% of participants conformed at least once, and 25% of participants never conformed. That means a quarter of us (or, a quarter of men?) can be counted on to speak the truth, even when the stooges decide in advance what is right or wrong.

So, what happened? During follow-up interviews, most said that they did not really believe their conforming answers. But, they had gone along with the group for fear of being ridiculed or thought "*peculiar*".

A few of them said that they really did believe the group's answers were correct. Eek.

Apparently, people conform for two main reasons: because they want to fit in with the group (normative influence) and because they believe the group is better informed than they are (informational influence).

In a world of too many obvious wrongs, what can help us expand that crucial quarter of men? Let your imagination wander now, to what you might think of the character of those 25% who resisted, having watched the scene play out, and knowing what you know about the variables. Would you feel admiration? Trust? Would you have considered them trouble-makers or truth-tellers? Is there a difference? Then, what if the 25% were largely women?

What if this unique kind of Not Caring What People Think could be a force of salvation in current North American culture?

This is an important skill in advancing any social change because opposition to you and your ideas will be ever-present. It is all too common that insecure and fearful people will lash out at the messenger. Especially when your message challenges a status quo, it may rock some people to their core. People can say unkind things when they're scared. You must be able to endure this. We get to Not Caring What People Think by practice, and also by knowing ourselves truly.

Once we see and own our shortcomings, we are infinitely freer.

Knowing our weak places, where we still need to grow, actually increases our confidence. It allows us to withstand any negative feedback because we have something solid to gauge it against. In my twenties, I kept ducks (among other animals) on a piece of land, and people offered me duck sayings. So many duck sayings and proverbs. Here is one of my favorites:

If one person calls you a duck, don't worry about it.
If two people call you a duck, think about it.
If three people call you a duck, start looking for
tail feathers.

One of the many gifts of friendship is having a reliable mirror in which to see ourselves. Sure, one person's harsh, negative assessment can be a fluke. If it's something we hear a lot from people close to us (not those who might be threatened by our message), then it deserves a closer look. The best connections give us even more courage to brave those darker places, with strength and resilience.

So, regardless of who may put us down, ask us to do wrong on their behalf, or pressure us to quietly go along... speaking the truth and Not Caring What People Think is always an option.

I care about my impact. I care about how my presence in people's lives affects their time in this world. I care about others' unique experiences and viewpoints. I care about the needs and feelings of others. In so many ways, I care deeply.

Certain people's opinions of me? Not my fucking business.

The Door Through Which You Came, The Second Door

At the time, and this is painful yet important to say, my parents pretended to not know what had happened. My brother Damon graduated in 1994 and was largely unaware. I learned many, many years later, that Steve Hahn had simply made phone calls to both fathers - with no written records saved or sent. Sybil's father got a phone call, as did mine. My parents spoke not a word about this to me. I didn't have the trust or confidence in them to seek out support. It had never really been like that.

I was clearly going nowhere at Acton-Boxboro, despite the wild fun I was having going there. So, I needed to attend summer school to pass the 11th grade. I actually remember that experience fondly. I enjoyed the condensed format of the many-hour-long sessions and the efficiency of it all. It crossed my mind more than once: could I just do the rest of it this way? The English class was far superior to the one offered in Acton, too. So, I added another insight into my expanding view of education. Summer school covered junior year.

Then came the choice for my last year.

Those days, I lived a funny tension right on the brink of actually disappearing (my parents knew this all too well) and psychologically and emotionally shutting down. There was a wild, defiant freedom in this, since I now had a driver's license and a car, which I'd bought with my own money from working at the horse barn. I had nearly everything I needed. It could all tip either way at any time.

My parents seemed to sense this and moved cautiously. Without my input, they began to plead with Lawrence Academy to let me back in for my senior year. I do remember learning of their pleading. I don't remember having a vote or being engaged at all in the matter. I would turn 18 in December, so the countdown was on. I could graduate or not. This was not my concern. One way or another, I was going, west and far away.

In the fall, I sat again in that same big, headmaster's office with a rotund, slow-moving man named Terry Murdoch. When I walked back through the door, I was all discernment and caution. I saw their dark side and would not be fooled or convinced otherwise. Blake was gone, graduated and off to college in New Hampshire. A number of my closest friends were gone. Some remained.

Mr. Murdoch would become my advisor, if I was permitted reentry. So, we sat in the office and bargained. I remember it being cloudy. There was a fog on everything. This was the early signs of shutting down. He laid out special restrictions (what restrictions did Pete Regis live under?, I wondered). I would not be allowed to leave campus during the day. This seemed funny, as I would soon be a legal adult. I would be a day student, of course. No one dared suggest I live on campus.

I wonder if it's clear here, just how thick the implication of blame was in that moment. These are the "micro-aggressions" that are meant to keep people in subordinate places. Every one of these steps gave a message that I was somehow the problem. Now, everywhere I looked, adults fell off the edge of right and wrong at great speed - and I finally did shut down. The fog descended. If they were trying to quiet my dissent, it was going to take a sleight of hand in reasserting dominance over my objections. I was done. My soul retreated as I entered the bottleneck that would eventually shoot me out and away from all of this.

I was a student at Lawrence Academy for my senior year, while Pete

Regis roamed the campus without consequence. Shutting down and armoring up are partners in the dance of not-feeling. Either one can lead at a given time. If I was going to be safe during my days on campus, I would not really be present. The vitality in me was gone, on reserve for another time. I kept myself physically off-campus as much as possible, too. Living through that year gave me enough of a taste of stifling under another's oppression, that I would never want to tolerate it again.

~ ~ ~

In order to survive, I began a few special rituals.

First, I spent hours and hours writing lists. These were my truest moments of joy that year, aside from the times when Sybil and I would join with new friends and have adventures. My heart opened to some new young people. But privately, I was planning my escape. I wrote out the food I would buy, diagram how to pack clothes into my car, and itemize tools I would need. A few friends knew of my plans, and even got caught up in the excitement, saying they wanted to come with me. One by one, they each fell away, though. Their parents said no. Or, they made other plans. These friends didn't seem to understand it wasn't frivolity for me. It was a survival plan.

The second ritual fed my soul in a time when the darkness of the untrustworthy adult world threatened to blot out the sun all around me.

I would wake before sunrise, hop in the car and drive to the coast of southern New Hampshire in the dark. There, on an eastern shore, I would begin walking before dawn and fully take in the slow rising of the sun. Barefooted and silent, I would move blissfully for as long as I could walk. I came to love that experience so much, the fulfillment of the brightened day was often a let down. I wanted it again.

I wanted to live in that magical space of darkness changing to light. It was the best I could do to evoke the knowing of things getting better. By meeting the sunrise over and over, I started to believe that life was more than silencing and corruption. Of course, it was. It had to be. I just hadn't seen it yet. The sunrise was so plain and real and undeniable, as it illuminated everything without fail. '*Again,*' my heart ached, '*again!*'.

I also didn't want it to end, because it meant I had to drive back to Massachusetts and face all that awaited me there.

Gramma and Grandpa came again in 1996. But everything was different this time. So little good could truly reach me anymore. Then, one day in May, my Grandfather suffered an aneurism. He was 84 at the time, and the trip to the hospital and his end all blurred into one grey and heavy smear on my life. He'd fallen off his chair a few weeks earlier, and I heard Gramma calling to me for help.

"Nessa! Nessa, honey, are you there?"

Their room was across the hall from mine.

"Daddy fell and we can't get him back up."

She called him Daddy, which I loved, because it made me think of how, once their sons were born, he was simply a daddy now. It was a statement of fully embracing the transition they made, from young lovers to parents. I walked in, and my Grandfather, who was hunched over with Parkinson's disease, lay awkwardly on the ground.

I knew how to lift with my legs and keep my back straight. When I reached my arm around his chest, I was amazed at how thin and slippery his soft skin was on his bones. This once-stately, gentle man barely ever spoke. He just looked at Gramma with a twinkle in his eye and said so many things with his presence alone. In this moment, though, he stammered, "Now, don't hurt yourself". Then, once we'd gotten him back up in his chair, Gramma swooned and sighed with relief. Grandpa spoke to me a second time. He said, "Thank you", his voice growing dry and crackly from strain, "Thank you... for saving our lives".

It was a profound thing to say, and I felt the warmth in his words. His eyes were brown and softened from age. He was from Spain and Gramma had always referred to him as swarthy. I knew him only in his softened, stooped, and radiantly warm, older state.

Then, just a few weeks later, he was gone. I had never lost anyone to death before, and here it was. In yet another layer of fog, I attended my first funeral at 18. My love and care for Gramma swelled as I watched her move through immense sadness, to somehow have the courage to keep going herself. They'd been married almost fifty years. The world was already grey, and then Grandpa slipped away from us.

~ ~ ~

Somehow and just barely, I graduated from high school. I had a few new friends, and a few old. I've heard it said that love makes all things bearable. My connection to them stays with me as I look back. I also remember that the school gave my younger sister a special award at my graduation. They called her up and had everyone clap. Somehow, that seemed one more subtle jab. It was a reminder that they rewarded students who, unlike me, obeyed and did not challenge their authority.

Well, as soon as ceremonies were over, I lit up a cigarette, right there on the campus quad. Ok, well, fuck you, too, then. It was finally time to go.

Right before setting out for the west coast, I had a dream about my Grandfather. He came to me and stood as easy and tall as I could imagine him. His voice was clear, too. Those things were different, but his warm, quiet way was exactly the same. He approached me gently, and said, "Be true to yourself."

Ok, Grandpa. I'll do my best.

~ ~ ~

It was early July when I finally went.

In the days leading up to my departure - it was a known date, and no secret to my parents - strange tensions were mounting in the house. My mother had been a portrait photographer in Chelmsford, a higher-functioning alcoholic, and largely absent from my childhood. Like I said, her swooping-in gestures were always swift, sudden and corrective. She tried to make me something I was not. I resisted. Then, she was gone.

In the momentum of all my preparations, my mother suddenly became fixated on wanting to take my portrait. As if all of her time spent drinking and absent from my care could be made up for in this moment. As if she could capture a false semblance of normalcy one last time. I am sure she was feeling a lot. But, I had a tight schedule and I was not pausing all of my focus now to accommodate her needs. She had always made it about her.

Those portrait sessions had been especially soul-stealing throughout my childhood. It involved make-up and excessive attention to hair. It involved sitting in forced, uncomfortable positions and making faces I would never, naturally make. It was the epitome of her trying to sculpt me into an image that fit her vision. It was not about truly seeing me. It was about her pretending I was what she had hoped and that she had succeeded.

There was absolutely no way I was doing this now.

Finally, we had a fight where all of the tensions peaked. She would not accept that I refused to participate in this. She was frantic. I was furious. I needed her to stop. It started in my room, and then, I was running through the house, screaming that I would not have her take my portrait. In my angst, I ran through the halls, into the kitchen, and her soaring anxieties followed me. I sailed down the stairs, at 18 years old and many inches taller than her. I was fast. Soon, I made it to the back door.

This door was 90% plate glass, with a wooden frame and a simple lever handle that had long ceased working. A "storm door", as New Englanders called it. We had always just kicked the base of the door open as we headed out to the backyard. The sound of us kids kicking it open and it shutting behind us was part of the soundtrack to our summers. It was how that house breathed.

So, I turned the corner at great speed and headed for the exit. I went to kick the wooden doorframe, like I'd done thousands of times before. Only I kicked too high. With the force of my momentum behind me, I couldn't stop moving as I heard the sound of breaking glass, splintering sharp in my ears. This glass was not tempered but shattered in great shards and daggers around me as I passed. I was running, soaring, right through the glass door.

The silence after all the pieces crashing down seemed to ripple out in waves. I breathed in and out. I checked my body for damage and gasped at the implausibility of it all. I had busted out, right through the door, and was miraculously, mostly ok.

~ ~ ~

Talk about barely getting out unscathed. I left for the west coast a few days later, with only a few scratches on my arm.

Departures

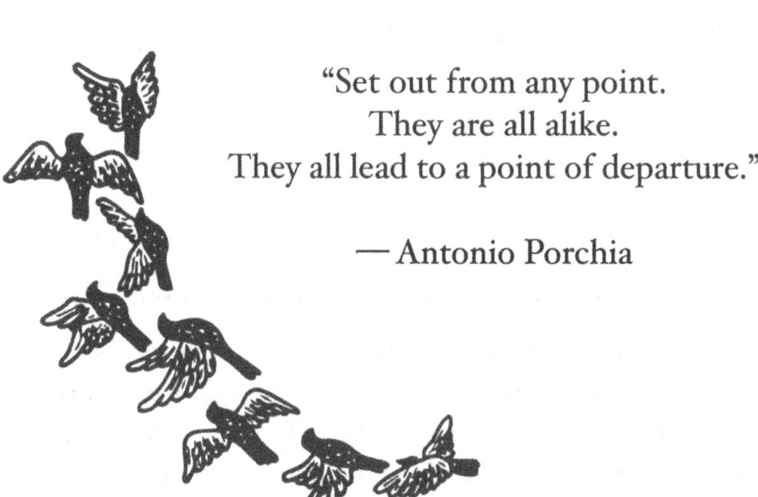

"Set out from any point.
They are all alike.
They all lead to a point of departure."

— Antonio Porchia

On the Road

"Better to sleep in an uncomfortable bed free,
than sleep in a comfortable bed unfree."

— Jack Kerouac

The road was a fine companion in a number of ways. For one, it gave me time to think, to calm my system, and gain insights that could only be found through long stretches of silence. I could cry or rage, wallow in despair, or find complete ecstasy in all the possibility that lay before me, and the road held it all. The steady hum of the engine and the rumbling of tires on pavement were like the soothing downbeat to all of the cacophonous storms moving within me. It was steady and reliable, like a true mirror to my own soul within the larger soul of the world.

As I set my own rhythms to that of whirling landscapes, cities, and plains, I found an increasing sense of calm and relief along the interstates. It didn't really matter where I was going, just that I was finally on my way. That momentum carried me a great, many, many miles.

I recall meeting a young man while passing through Arizona and telling him I was traveling without destination. He said, "Hopefully, you have a great stereo system in that car.". I said, "Actually, I haven't turned on the radio for maybe three days, now." He was shocked. How blissfully the silence helped to cleanse me of all I'd seen.

When the storms in my heart receded, I would inevitably rest into running the fingers of my memory over threads of connection in love with people I'd known back east. I had time to ponder our connection, what it was to me, all that was given and received. The heart, like an instrument, grows more resonant and intricate with the strumming of finely-tuned strings.

I still held a belief in the goodness of humanity, and I needed evidence of those different ways to live. I needed to see places and relationships where other values and priorities were honored and expressed. I was awaiting the fulfillment of that faith I'd cultivated along the beach in southern New Hampshire. I had to feel the movement of other winds animating this life.

The road provided.

Since my early goal was to go as far as I could, for as long as I could, I ate simply and sparsely (lots of bananas and peanut butter) and slept in my car at night. I would tuck my long hair into a blue, trucker-style ARCO baseball cap and hide any evidence of my being female. By evening, I'd crawl in back, tuck myself under drab grey blankets, and nestle in to sleep. I had a number of steeds over the years - many Volkswagons, occasionally a Toyota truck (those were the days!).

I learned to become a connoisseur of parking lots. Rest stops always gave me the heebie-geebies, so other locales became my resting places. Motel parking lots offered an ideal mix of companionable human activity and anonymity. The people running them, and the people traveling through, expected cars with out-of-state license plates to be in their lots. So, it was a great form of cover. Church parking lots were sweet in a pinch, with a higher risk for the "Can I help you?" question, yet more solitude and true quiet. Any night but Saturday night, this was a good option.

I traveled in the days before cell phones when you could actually find $.78/gallon for regular unleaded in the deep south. In the early years of criss-crossing the country, I stuck to the Interstates. Wide, steady roads of many lanes, sturdy and very well-traveled. It took maybe four or five times of reaching the coast before I felt comfortable enough to leave that security and venture onto the minor roads, the "Blue Highways", as William Least-Heat Moon calls them. Then, I really got to know this country.

There is the America that is advertised to those moving through quickly. You'll know our commerce and our superficial values through the imagery of billboards and quick-pull-off, full-service stations. Then, there is the America that actually breathes the heart and soul of this land - those places that still echo the diverse cultures and stories of how it all became inhabited. That soul holds the hope and pain, the tragedy, and the enduring human kindness that all great endeavors do. I was enchanted to experience so many subcultures. I still value this about the country, with a unique personality and landscape to every region.

I especially loved how the land began to show up in the faces of those I met. I could see the resemblance. It was like learning a new language, just in meeting so many people and lands in rapid succession. I saw these intricacies in motion, like doing flashcards of, 'How does the human being wear the midwest/the mid-Atlantic/etc.?'. I still love to study a face and see if I can recognize a land in the expressions and look in the eyes. We become what we love, and the mark of that love soon shows itself on both.

~ ~ ~

During my first stay in California, I took a proper Automotive class at Sierra College, in the dry, north-central region, so I could feel more competent traveling long-distances alone. There was one other young woman in the class, and a lot of respectful, rugged guys all focused on learning the trade. I could change a flat tire, do an oil change, and even repair a brake system with help. I recall traveling I-5 in the Northwest and seeing an elderly couple pulled over beside the left, fast lane of the freeway. The white-haired man was hunched, but fit, and trying to perform some repair. I pulled off at the next exit and made my way south again. I saw them still struggling. Then, I pulled back onto the northbound and slowly pulled up behind them.

This man looked to be about 80, clean-cut and humble. His wife, also white-haired, was nervous and kind. They were trying to change a flat. I told them about my automotive class and, would they please let me help them? I tried to pose it as a game I enjoyed, to see how quickly I could do it. I knew a man of that generation would be hesitant to relinquish his task to a young woman. But, in sweet relief, he relented. I got that tire changed in under ten minutes, and they were beaming with gratitude. Then, we were all on our way.

Most of my time was simple east-west travel, with the intention to just not repeat already-traveled roads. All told, I would cross the country, coast-to-coast, twelve times, visiting all 48 contiguous states and parts of Canada. My higher education on the actual "real world" surpassed most of what school had provided. During these moving meditations, I would feel into which direction to turn, with luscious hundreds of miles to choose from, and find the experiences I most needed to meet.

This practice was a sweet experiment in surrender. I had always been so over-responsible, caring for my younger siblings, and looking out for others at the school. I always felt that I needed to step up and protect and do what others could not. In those years, it was medicine for my soul to just ask the larger forces around me to direct me. On the road, I got to be a child of something much bigger than all of us. I felt I was floating along the surface of a glorious river. I grew to love that river, and it still runs along the veins of my life. Like a current I can dip my fingers into anytime life's unfolding grows dry or brittle, I feel it there. We met when I was bright, youthful, and seeking renewal. It still informs my choices.

I believe we all enter this world with unique gifts and are forever guided toward their discovery and expression. Once we remove all pressures to meet others' expectations or fulfill "success" on unimportant terms, we are reliably moved where we most need to be. There was ecstasy in moving with it then, and most of all, in being moved.

There were places, though, I knew of and had to reach for personal reasons. So, in 1998, I was headed to New Orleans. My Spanish Grandfather had roots in the city, his ancestors being Creole among the rich cultural blend on the bayou. I had such a strong feeling when Gramma talked about it. So, I needed to see what I could discover there, of the lineage and bloodline through such a fabled place.

~ ~ ~

On my way, my 1976 Volkswagon broke down after dark, on a country road outside the town of Opelousas, Louisiana. I couldn't sleep in the car on that little road with no shoulder. I had to set out on foot. I closed the car door behind me, checking for my AAA membership, and tuned in to a deeper knowing as I wandered out into the night. I was listening to my instincts, focusing on what I needed to accomplish.

I saw in the distance the warm glow of a porch light through the trees. Most of the homes on that road had a good five to ten acres of land around each one. So, the lights of houses were few. I approached one and took in all the visual information. I listened to my body and sensed the quality of all I was encountering in the darkness. Soon enough, I could hear two middle-aged women sitting on a porch in dim light, talking.

As I approached, the quality of their voices sounded kind and familiar. They were having a very uneventful evening and casually sharing it together. I decided to make my presence known with my voice first, so I wouldn't startle them as I appeared from the darkness. I called out in announcement and question, "Hello," as I walked into view. I told them I had broken down, and may I use their phone? They agreed, seeming slightly concerned about the 19-year-old on their porch. They offered me some iced tea to accompany my phone call.

The tow truck driver on the line said he would meet me by the Volkswagon within the hour. Soon, a large man with a booming voice and jovial presence approached me at the side of the road. He asked where I was headed, and I said, New Orleans. He asked where he wanted me to take the car. I had a AAA Plus membership, with 100 miles of free towing. So I figured, if I was that close, he could just take me there and suggested it.

Then, he said, "Darlin, there is no way in hay-yell I am taking you and your broken down car to New Orleans at this hour.". He said, "Look, my wife and I live right here on Main Street in Opelousas, and sometimes we take in people when they come into trouble, and give them a place stay until it blows over." I admitted I'd been sleeping in my car as I traveled around the country.

"Now, if you're sleeping in your car, that's your right, and I won't stop you from doing it at our local service station. So, you can think about it. But, if you decide that it suits you, Nancy and I would love to have you at our home. We have a 17-year-old daughter, too, who would be real excited to meet you." All of my instincts told me this was a solid, kind, and safe human being. While I was slightly disappointed to not make it to New Orleans yet, I agreed. Round about midnight, I walked onto their front porch and into their home with the spare room. There, I stretched out flat on a full-sized bed and slept.

I stayed with this family a whole week, a number of days longer than it took for the mechanic to patch the electrical system on the Volkswagon. They also ran the General Store in town, so I'd spend my days with their 17-year old daughter, sitting on tall stools eating snacks, and chatting with the locals. Looking back now, I think they were flattered that I would give their little town an extended stay, as if my choice gave merit to its charms as a tourist attraction.

I braided Nancy's hair in the morning on Sunday before church services. I told her I had an interest in real gospel music and asked if their church sang the gospel. She said they'd sing a hymn here and there. She asked me, "Do you believe in God?". I replied, "I believe in *a* god.". She did her best in her southern hospitality to hide her shock and dismay. I did not attend services that day. Instead, the daughter and I walked the rounds of Main Street while I learned all about her life.

I always preferred to leave any place I had stayed a while, during the dark hour before sunrise. Perhaps it was a continuation of that old ritual of walking the southern coast of New Hampshire in the dark to light time. The warmth of the expanding sunlight was such a reassurance to me. My kinship with that sacred hour encouraged me toward whatever-came-next. One day, in an idle moment, Nancy said to me optimistically, "Maybe you'll meet your husband in Opelousas, and settle down here." I was gone the next morning, with a Thank You note and another sunrise to send me on my way.

~ ~ ~

In New Orleans, I found even more enchantment and cultural richness than I imagined. The heavy air hung on the moss dripping from stately old trees, and the arts scene was so thick with music, it seemed to pour out of every corner. I felt the potent Creole lineage in the magic shops, where voodoo was a way of life, far more authentic than any suspicious movie reference. The people and the land had a thousand stories to tell me, and every one drew me closer in to a sense of home, and further out toward a feeling of adventure in exotic lands.

The city seemed to regard me in a similar way. So many of my encounters were with people I would describe as 'juicy', just dripping with a warm love of life, one that wanted to cock its head to a side and proclaim, "Well, ain't you the *cutest*?". New Orleans was luscious. I soaked up the shameless way the residents embraced color, vitality, oozing artistic expression, all with a sultry drawl of people just living the poetry of life. Even now, I recall that pre-Hurricane-Katrina New Orleans with a scrumptious heart swell of affection.

I ran out of money there and worked at the youth hostel to pay my stay. It was an easy rhythm of shifts, and downtime spent out in the courtyard with fellow travelers. I remember a man at the hostel asked me to marry him. It seemed to me a lot of people had marrying on the mind in Louisiana. As if there was something like an unfinished sentence about a woman of 19 traveling alone. Maybe in the south, it was just hard to imagine that "A woman of 19 travels alone." was a complete sentence.

One night, I wandered out to see what fun I could find in the French Quarter on foot. Partway there, a man of about 25 pulled over on a motorbike and started speaking to me in hushed tones. Instinctively, he felt like one of my brothers or an old guy friend from high school to whom I could tell anything. He said, "I don't mean to startle you, but I saw you walking by. Then, I saw a man starting to follow you and gain pace quickly in a not-cool way. This isn't the best neighborhood to be walking in after dark. If you'll trust me, I can give you a ride on my bike to wherever it is you are going." I looked down the sidewalk from where I came and did see a figure moving quickly toward us in the distance. I looked into this young man's eyes. I hopped on.

As we moved through the humid air, the coolness of the breeze making the sensation so pleasant, I told him I was heading into the French Quarter. He laughed, as if to say, "Of course." I told him I did travel in from far away. He asked if there was anything else I wanted to see on our way there. Now, he was both a proud savior and tour guide; he was on his way into the French Quarter, too. We both relaxed into the ease of the ride. I talked about my grandfather having lived in the city, and wondered, "Where could I find those bizarre, above-ground cemeteries?". I wanted to look for relatives with the same Spanish last name. We cruised along the levies on the city's edge, and he pointed toward the best area to explore in the morning.

He took me into intricate, lively streets of the French Quarter, bringing me into bars where I normally wouldn't have been given entry, as a 19-year old. He was a friendly young local, and the regulars all smiled a warm smile to see him. Cody was his name. He introduced me around, and I felt even more at ease with an ally to help me enjoy this remarkable place. He dropped me off at the hostel at the end of the night, with absolute gentlemanly southern charm.

The next day, I wandered those cemeteries on foot, where the water was an even larger presence than the land. I was enchanted to find a few "Fatjo" name markers among them - the true spelling of my Spanish last-name, signaling the torch-makers of long ago.

I left New Orleans too early, before sunrise one day. A horrible flu had overtaken me. I was broke and sick, and I had been on the road for a month or more. I decided it was time to go back to Massachusetts to see what kind of replenishment I could find there. My stops back east in the early days were focused and brief. Each one included a stop into Steve Hahn's office to tend this unaddressed risk to kids. Always, I hoped my consistent push would be enough to knock them out of complacency.

For the first seven years, my visits were roughly annual. After that, they soon dwindled to none at all. Addressing the issue at Lawrence Academy gave me purpose, but seeking rejuvenation with my family always proved futile. Even when something isn't good for you, sometimes it takes a few rounds of away and back, away and back again, until we're finally ready to let it go.

~ ~ ~

I had nothing but good fortune, and even protection, in my time traveling the country alone by car. One time, I broke down on Interstate 5 in the Northwest (long before I would call it home). I pulled over, not knowing how far it was to the nearest off-ramp. Remember, this was before cell phones - or, a time when they were rare enough that pay phones were still common in every town. So, I took a marker and some chipboard from a box of crackers and drew out the old, universal symbol for a phone. I tucked my hair up into my baseball hat and put on my baggiest clothing: a hoodie and straight-legged corduroys. I stood by the side of the road and my car, holding out the phone symbol.

Soon, a car did pull over. I approached slowly to the passenger-side window and found a woman of about 60 in the driver's seat. When she rolled down the window to speak, her first words were, "Oh, I thought you were a boy standing there.". *Success!*, I thought. She rapidly followed with, "Honey, don't you ever do that again!" in a tone of exasperation. She felt compelled to scold me for being a woman on the side of the road, asking for help in broad daylight. I borrowed her phone, and soon after, a AAA-dispatched tow truck came and brought me and my car to the nearest town.

The thing I learned most from the road was this:

You find what you put out there.

I definitely encountered the many people who would say, "Aren't you worried about axe-murderers and psychopaths?". That was the phrasing of time, in the late 1990s. I said I wasn't. I believed there was good in the world, and I was determined to find it. I noticed, the more I put that thought and intention into the world, the more quickly I would encounter it.

I needed to know I could be in this world and determine the safe people from the unsafe people. I was reorienting myself toward a new ability to discern and trust. The hardest thing was having bought the story that Lawrence Academy of Groton, Massachusetts, was not only a safe place but a superior place for the wellbeing of young people. I accepted that story without question as a 14-year old - and it had been the grandest of lies. So, I needed to reset my inner compass to ensure that I would be able to detect disturbances in the frequency between what was said and what was true. I could tune my perceptions to a deeper truth, beneath the words written or spoken, and arrive at my own conclusion. I could steer through this world, with all of its deceptions and illusions, and still know what was safe.

The closest I ever came to an unsettling situation was one evening, sleeping in a sparsely-filled parking lot. I had learned to always place the car near enough to a street light to discourage trouble, but far enough that I wouldn't be easily seen sleeping inside. So, I was awakened in the night by headlights streaming by and a loud, rumbling engine breaking the silence. I carefully watched from my inside camp and saw a ragged mini-van pass me by, then slowly circle back around my car. It got my heart racing. But, I knew how to instantly drop into my instinctual listening. From there, I only sensed the subtle intrigue of bored teenagers with little to do. Of course, I couldn't see who was driving - and I made sure they couldn't see me. Then, I watched them slowly drive away.

It called to mind Amazing Grace, "through many dangers, toil, and snares, I have already come..." Maybe it was all the middle America church radio.

~ ~ ~

The peak experience of my road-tripping days came in a way I didn't expect.

There was a moment of arrival that I couldn't have anticipated and didn't see coming. It wasn't a geographical arrival, but a sense of peace where I had convinced myself that I was safe. I could do it. That no matter what I encountered, true or false, ill-intended or good, I was going to be ok. And it wasn't just my own internal practice of listening to my instincts. It was a larger sense that something greater than me would look out for my wellbeing if I surrendered to it.

It happened on the very windy plains of west Texas. I remember a number of times over the years, I would run low on gas in the night - and arrive at a gas station after dark to find it closed. I didn't have the fuel to get back on a highway and keep seeking another gas stations. Logical common sense told me if this one was closed, the next one would be too. So, I spent many nights parked at various gas stations, waiting for them to open the following day.

I had driven quite a ways through this straight, flat, open plain in Texas, only to find that the gas station was no longer a gas station. It was closed, as in, closed for good a long time ago. I had probably driven across the country three or four times at this point. If you think of it as a career, of instinct and safety-navigation-training, I wasn't brand new on the job. But I had paid some dues. It wasn't a novel experience anymore, driving across the country. There was so much yet to explore and so many new ways to experience it.

So, I remember the feeling as I pulled into this gas station, with a sweet lack of tension in any of it. Maybe at that point, I'd already cultivated such a sense of trust in this thing that keeps me moving, keeps me going, and keeps me safe. You could say I felt its presence in a reassuring way. I slept in my car by an old, abandoned gas station, so exposed to the sky and the vast expanse in all directions. No trees, or extra structures, just an expanse lay out before and all around me. There was no angst in me even as I went to sleep that night. I felt fully at ease as I drifted off in my familiar back seat camp.

In the morning, I was awakened by the movement of the whole car, shaking back and forth in the wind. The little Volkswagon was rocking side to side with the force of winds from so far away, and it was so good. It's hard to find the words, though it brings up my love for the wind in general. When I awoke in that little car being shaken by the winds of west Texas, I felt utter confidence that nothing would hurt me.

For the first time, I relaxed into the feeling that I could be held by something other than a family structure, or a house, by a school structure or its dorms. I had mapped out, by connect-the-dots, this interconnected current of movement and synchronicity across the landmass. I saw I had an active role in it: being conscious of what I believed, and how that would be shown to me. You find what you put out there. I was allowed to be scared in moments, and I could trust myself to not succumb to that fear. I would acknowledge it and then take a different road. These pathways were as vast as the country itself, and they would hold me safe, even rock me like a baby in their arms.

I was giddy with the joy. The exhilaration of being safe in a windstorm in the middle of nowhere and all was still more than well. I was riding and being rocked by it, my own bucking bronco of a car in the wind. I could relax and laugh and feel so alive. I had become the leaf on the river's surface, no matter what the current. This feeling was so real that it reset my system, almost completely, for the first time.

The Body Speaks - 2001

"Some patients discover their own islands of safety - this sets the stage for trauma resolution: pendulating between states of exploration and safety, between language and body."

— Bessel van der Kolk, MD

In the year 2001, seven years after running away from home, my body started to speak up. I had been returning to Massachusetts and Lawrence Academy every year since to stop into Steve Hahn's office and address the situation. That situation being: they were sheltering a child molester on campus, and I knew about it. In 1997, I attended my sister's high school graduation and saw Pete Regis as the first face greeting families on campus. He was directing traffic and welcoming families on foot. Steve and I had a talk that year after ceremonies. Then, I wrote him letters from my new home in Berkeley, California.

Each year, with each new visit, there was a new false promise. Steve sat down with me each time, but always for the end-goal of convincing me everything was fine. I know now it was also a kind of risk-mitigation. If he could convince me he cared and might do something, then legal repercussions were less likely. I didn't know it at the time, but there was a statute of limitations at play: they had seven years to dodge me and avoid being sued. Just seven years. So, if he could deflect me for that long, he might hide his horrible choice eternally. The thought of suing the school never occurred to me once, alarmed as I was at the ongoing threat to new students.

Of course, every one of those encounters impacted me as a personal insult. Each time this man failed to act on my concerns, it gave me the message that what Sybil and I had endured was insignificant. Steve Hahn was so comfortable, after all. He was smug and unmoving, even while he spoke empty words of concern and agreement. He was two people right before my eyes: the one who presented as if he cared, and the one blithely risking kids' safety. He was employing the same kind of trickery Pete Regis had. Steve Hahn was abusing his power in a way that misleads.

This is the early rumblings of corruption. When someone seeks to mislead you while protecting their comfort, you have entered the terrain of intentional off-steadying . . .

So now, a new kind of distress kept me up at night. Whether I was living in some town on the west coast or traveling on the road, it visited as a nagging, wildly-urgent awareness. I was learning how to tend my own safety, but the longevity of that unacceptable situation grew unbearable. My years of insistence to Steve Hahn started adding up to a new kind of panic for me. All those times I had gathered my strength to walk onto campus again, the confrontation with Pete Regis receding into the distance, became insignificant without any results to follow. I was doing all I could think to do, while Pete was waiting to lure one more student into his garage, all under Steve Hahn's watch. Because I knew, I was painfully now, complicit. The tragedy of things going unchanged for so long started eating me up inside.

~ ~ ~

In 2001, I was living in rural Bayside, California, between the towns of Eureka and Arcata, CA. The "bay" in Bayside referred to Humboldt Bay, and this town was a lovely stretch of sloughs and grey wetlands with white egrets, linking the two small towns. Everywhere I lived in Humboldt County,

California, I could see horses from my window. I had a wonderful partner then, and we had moved in together at the beginning of the year. At 23 years old, this was a big step for me. We were easy with one another and fell into a sweet rhythm of school, working, gardening together, and sharing adventures on the town. I was smoothly content there, feeling free, and enjoying the love of a good man.

Then, suddenly, my body started speaking up. I was taking Women's Studies classes at Humboldt State University, a small state school nestled in the redwoods on a hill above Arcata. Amidst studies in ecology and environmental resource engineering, I discovered the social justice issues of gender and power. Suddenly, the world opened up to me. I believe this insight into the context of my life is what seriously got my body's attention.

Suddenly, all that I had endured at Lawrence Academy of Groton, Massachusetts, fit succinctly into this much larger political story of struggle and triumph. The silencing efforts by an elite and over-paid male staff at an old-boy institution were only a continuation of historical oppressions leading up to the present-day. I could now see and name the threads of injustice that wove all around my personal experience: sexism, elitism, patriarchy, and classism. The weaving of threads was just the right metaphor, too. Suddenly, I was having intense abdominal pain that had no real explanation.

I went in for ultrasounds and learned there was a mass on my right ovary. It made for pain in ways I'd never experienced. It was no coincidence that this also was the year my efforts with Lawrence Academy reached a peak. The day arrived as suddenly as the pain in my belly. I had undergone a laparoscopic surgery that summer, with the sweetest Planned Parenthood employee, and my partner by my side. I'd never had factual information about my body - let alone reverent, celebratory information. An older woman named Madeline went above and beyond by choosing to accompany me clear through this process.

I remember her going over ultrasound photos with me and gushing at how beautiful my organs were. Her sweet and bold spirit was similar to that of my grandmother. She said to my partner of me, "There's just something about her honest nature that captures my heart.". By some blessing of circumstances, I had a great partner and a loyal, loving woman to accompany me on this frightening experience of learning about 'the mass'.

Now, the most amazing thing was what happened during surgery. The mass had been palpable, measurable, and very clear in shape and size on the ultrasound. The pain to let me know of its existence was also undeniable. Then, the night before surgery, I had a strange nightmare...

> *I dreamt I was frantically running through a war-torn scene, all sand-yellow tones and tent-like structures strewn about from whatever devastation had come through. There were some people around, just barely keeping themselves together. I was calling for my mother, and even though I knew she was there, it was clear in the dream that she was choosing to ignore me. Of course, I didn't understand why.*

I woke up with my heart thumping in my chest and nearly sweating. I felt I'd visited some very real and ancient hell that somehow lived in my body's memory. I was scared. Going under anesthesia, while an unknown mass is removed from the tender center of your body, is absolutely vulnerable. I had wonderful support. But, the journey was ultimately mine to take alone.

So, I arrived at the local Eureka, California, hospital that morning. I don't remember all the steps, but I felt safe and well-cared-for. When I awoke, Madeline was there to talk me through what they found. She said, "Honey, we can't explain it, but the mass was gone." "Gone?" I asked. It had just been there. "Yes, I know. All they can think is, it must have burst and reabsorbed. We believe it was fluid-filled, but they didn't have to remove it.". I was amazed and somehow happily surprised at my body's defiant change of plans.

Then she said, "They did find some endometriosis, and cauterized it.". That was a new word and the beginning of a new adventure. Endometriosis can present as a weaving of fibrous threads all around the reproductive system. Still, about that mass! How mysterious that it would show up to get me in, focused on taking care of my body, and then be on its way now that I was showing up to listen. That experience began a new kind of practice for me, of listening. I slowly became very attuned to what my belly, my ovaries, and all of my body were telling me in any given situation.

Then, many weeks post-surgery, a different kind of surprise arrived in the mail.

Ask & You Shall Receive, Part One

It was a sunny, late summer day in Northern California. I was feeling stronger and fully recovered from surgery with the mysterious, disappearing mass. I walked the lovely gravel road to the cluster of mailboxes at the end of our path. It was quiet and still, the way it always was on the tranquil lane that ended in a field of blackberries by the mailboxes.

I reached into the mailbox and pulled out what felt like an artifact of an ancient civilization. It was a glossy newsletter from Lawrence Academy of Groton, Massachusetts.

Had they not gotten the memo? '*Don't ask this one for money.*'. Seven years later, and no one had ever tracked me down as a potential donor. Then, someone had. It was ludicrous that I would hold such a thing in my hands on a rural Northern California road, given my history. With an uneasy, discerning eye, I read it.

They were celebrating all the great things their kids had done, with photos of sports teams and group hugs. Boasting, middle-aged white men stood shaking hands with other white men, smiling over a monetary exchange. It felt like the brochure to a strange and foreign land, standing on my quiet, country road. I sat down on a ledge to browse...Then, I saw it.

"We are going to be asking alumni for their input on the school.".

Holy Fuck. That was me. And, oh, yes! I had things to say.

Something about them finding me all the way out there, all those years later, with that ridiculously self-congratulatory magazine just sent me over the edge. I instantly stomped down to my converted barn and called Steve Hahn. I was Done.

"What the hell was this?" I asked him. "I read the line about input from alumni - I have things to say!". I released every fiery expression of 'fuck this' that cared to surface from the depths of my being. They all had a turn. "You have blown me off too many times now. You have a fucking child molester on campus - and I know about it! I am going to write editorials to The Boston Globe, The Lowell Sun. I am NOT keeping quiet about this anymore.".

It's funny how life will often give us foreshadowings of our future that we can't even recognize at the time. Somewhere leading up to this moment, I had imagined myself giving a speech at Lawrence Academy. Of course, I had frustration. Imagination would have been necessary to keep going. Knocking on that highest door over and over again was not getting results. I still think it is worth knocking, as one part of change-making strategy. The decision-makers need to be made uncomfortable and aware. But, I could not count on Steve Hahn to do the right thing. Ever. He'd gotten himself very comfortable at my expense and others' risk - and I was fucking Done.

I don't remember all the details or what we accomplished in each phone call. I just knew I was insistent now, and one way or another, I was exposing them. I'd laid out options, and he had chosen. He called back sometime later with a date and a time for me to speak at the school.

In retrospect, it is funny how easily these men convinced themselves they would be able to control things. It is an Achillea's heel. They are over-confident that they can just say, 'So it is', and so it will be. Maybe that's one of the warning signs of privilege gone-sour. The illusion that one can expect others to do to their will, and it will be so, without question.

'Abraham, I want you to kill your son to please me'

'Alright, God, I'll do it.'

Steve Hahn agreed to let me come back to Lawrence Academy on December 10, 2001, because he believed he would be able to control what I would and would not say. If it was all risk-management, one speech might have been better than exposure in the newspapers. I imagine now, Steve Hahn probably had a conversation with the school's attorney after my phone call - and risks were weighed and assessed. Since they'd gotten so many kids and parents to be quiet about Pete Regis for so long, they were arrogant in their belief that they could procure silence once again.

So it was, we had a date set. Given the enormity of what I was about to do, of course, I would drive. I had a great Toyota pickup truck with a camper shell at this point, so the overnights would be easy. I could load up the back with wool blankets and be truly cozy for most, if not all, of the country. Never mind that it was December.

Ten days was always the quickest I believed one could drive across the country and minimally enjoy it. Truckers will tell you it can be done in three. But, I wasn't just hauling goods. I was composing, processing, and preparing. I needed the time and the gradually shifting landscape. I needed the road and all it offered me. So, by late November, I was packing up the Toyota with my wool blankets, notebooks, a mini-cassette recorder, and tiny tapes. I was on my way east.

Trauma - The Live Wire of Survival

There was a rhythm in my recovery process and my life all through those years. California was a brilliant place to run away to, for so many reasons. It was a land that had generated so many significant changes in our culture and politics as a nation. On a practical level, I could always find a small town that called to me. If it had a junior college, I could continue to accumulate credits slowly as I explored the world. Then, I would soon head out to travel the country by car again.

I was geographically pendulating across the country, from the place of original impact to safety, and back. I was learning to stay with it and building tolerance for revisiting both the feelings and the place. Trauma is its own departure. It is a momentary leave, where the body separates from the intensity of sensations for a time - until we become strong enough to integrate it.

The truth is, I couldn't stay long anywhere. Ten months became an average threshold. It was as if seeing the cycle of a year come to fruition was too big a commitment, or somehow too risky. I couldn't name what that risk was; I only felt it in my body. I finally knew something larger was at play when I first arrived in Eureka, California, in 1999.

It was the fourth region of California I would call home. There, I rented a charming one-story cottage in the redwoods. It sat in a line of three nearly identical cottages, with a path that led into an ancient forest beyond our shared driveway. The place was magical for me. I befriended my neighbors, and we would share bar-b-qs and fires under the stars. I even built a treehouse in a cluster of redwoods in my spare time, between classes at the junior college and my job at the Redwood Hostel north of town. It was there I met the man I would love and live with two years later, at 23.

My cottage in Eureka was the first space I ever had all to myself, beyond living in my cars. Living alone was a thrill initially. Being one of five kids always made personal space hard to find. Here, I was living alone and without a television for the very first time in my life. Up to that point, as an adult, I had roommates who always had a TV, one way or another. That may seem like a random detail - but it was crucial. There are so many ways to distract ourselves from ourselves. It's remarkable. Even the culturally-approved ways can create a separation from whatever we most need to feel and face. You may not even notice you are missing something.

Sometimes, the people I met in my travels would marvel at my courage to move around so freely and see the world. They would say things like, "You are so brave to travel by yourself like that.". Often, I would then quietly think to myself, '*Yet, I think you are so brave to stay!*'. With my own little house in Eureka, I was actually staying put. It was three years after leaving home that I first tried the novel experience. Then, things rose to the surface for me.

All relationships are this way. Whether it's the relationship to a place, a person, a job, or some personal endeavor - our old wounds will arise for revisiting once we stay put. It's what we do next that matters.

One night, many months into enjoying my new space, I was agitated and couldn't sleep. I got up out of bed and started pacing the floors of my beautiful cottage after dark. I knew I was upset but didn't understand why. I'd told the story of Lawrence Academy in good company earlier that day (as I was doing more often then), and hadn't realized how stirred up I'd been. I had this wild panic in my physiological system. Something was happening in my body. My heart was racing, and I was too agitated to even be still. I couldn't read a book on the sofa. I couldn't make tea or settle down. My senses were all heightened, and I was jumpy and unsettled. I found myself not sleeping and racing with some energy I could barely contain. I felt alive - only, too alive. I was touching the urge to survive, like the live-wire of a downed electrical line, flopping wildly in the wind and rain.

When that electricity came disconnected from its sturdy pole, it was an unruly force. When harnessed and connected in to something larger, it could fuel many great things.

But for me, in northern California that evening, something undeniable was happening that I couldn't explain. In the early years, the currents moving through that line would sometimes become too great, and my system would go into overload. Even the consciousness would change, and thoughts only streamed in as ways to secure survival. Soon, I concluded - with misplaced purpose and relief - that I could harness that energy into going. Once the energy had an outlet, I was more able to manage. I could sleep.

I started planning my escape.

I had spent too long in Massachusetts, feeling trapped. Most of all, I was traumatized by the loss of safety on the Lawrence Academy campus. When they allowed a child molester to stay after I confronted him, the ground slipped out from under me. It was all confusion and terror. The energy of that fear got stored in my body and started coming out in unexpected ways, as I tried to reenter normal life as a young adult. There was a pattern where my rattled system would go into overload, and the only way to resolve it was to go.

I did soon leave Eureka, California, yet with more sadness than any previous departure. The good news is, when it came time to stop driving around the country, I returned to the area again and found a new home in neighboring Bayside, California the following year. I returned to a familiar for the first time, and back then, that was progress.

I often say how a connection to the body's wisdom is the most reliable source of information. Yet, I do need to clarify here - when our bodies go into overload from post-traumatic stress or flashbacks, we can only really make sense of the messages again once we regain equilibrium. It takes a lot of awareness and practice to recognize and say to ourselves, 'Oh, I am in a trauma state, and this won't make sense again until my system calms back down.'.

Things like heart rate, dilation of pupils, blood sugar levels, hormonal fluctuations (flooding with stress hormones like adrenaline and cortisol) all contribute to overload. We can learn to work with these processes to regain equilibrium and recover more and more quickly from an overstimulated or triggered state. Once we understand the forces that move in us and in the world, we can learn to work with them in masterful ways.

I remember talking to a therapist on the east coast in 2006, a full decade after leaving home. I was getting antsy to go. I spoke of the urgency of going - yet again - and traveling west. She asked me what urged me so strongly to go that way. I said forcefully, "I am not going to live in fear.". The east coast and fear were still so intricately linked in my system.

She remarked on the charge behind that statement, and that charge still lives in me now. Once you know what it is to be trapped by fear, you can make a fierce commitment to not live under that bind again. The promise that sprang from that charge is just the power I've grown to appreciate in myself, knowing it was part of my salvation.

For me, that meant flinging myself as far as possible into an unknown - and knowing I could be safe within it.

Useful Skills - Willing to Piss People Off

"Being responsible sometimes means pissing people off."

— Colin Powell, On Leadership

Being Willing to Piss People Off flows directly from the earlier skill, Not Caring What People Think.

Once you release concerns over other peoples' opinions, pissing them off - for a good cause - becomes much more possible. This practice also calls into question the issue of loyalty. I've had to learn this many times, as I value loyalty deeply. Yet, there are shades of rightness in living by it. At times, we will have to be loyal to our principles above our commitment to a person or an organization. That's hard. If there is mutual commitment on all sides, we can become loyal to both inside a relationship. They are not mutually exclusive.

Doing the right thing will piss off the people who benefit from it being wrong. As Jen Hatmaker, author of *Fierce, Free and Full of Fire,* says, "Every lie is costing somebody something. Every single lie we are telling or protecting, maybe it's just in our silence that we're protecting a lie - but it is costing somebody something." She continues, "So, the question is, who is benefitting from this lie, and who's paying the price? Because it's never neutral. It is never neutral."

In the Lawrence Academy abuse cover-up situation, it was so clear who was benefitting and who was paying the price. It was time to rebalance the scales.

Our relationship with ourselves and our integrity is the heart of what we have. It is the most enduring thing we ever have in our lives. That relationship eventually defines the quality of all our closest relationships, and our lives in every way, beyond us.

For that relationship, we can risk pissing people off, enduring their retaliation or ridicule, and continue to speak truth all the same. If you are going to be true to yourself, there will be no getting around it.

In his book, *Originals*, Adam Grant describes the four basic options for handling a dissatisfying situation: Exit, Voice, Persistence, and Neglect. The findings are based on decades of research and outlined in a 1970 book by economist Albert Hirschman, "Exit, Voice and Loyalty".

"**Exit** - means removing yourself from the situation altogether - quitting a miserable job, ending an abusive marriage, or leaving an oppressive country.

Voice - involves actively trying to improve the situation - approaching your boss with ideas for enriching your job, encouraging your spouse to seek counseling, or becoming a political activist to elect a less-corrupt government.

Persistence - is gritting your teeth and bearing it - working hard, even though your job is stifling, sticking by your spouse, or supporting your government even though you disagree with it.

Neglect - entails staying in the current situation, but reducing your effort - doing just enough at work not to get fired, choosing new hobbies that keep you away from your spouse, or refusing to vote."

Everyone connected to the situation at Lawrence Academy had a response that fit into one of these categories.

"If you do feel you can make a difference, but you aren't committed to the person, country, or organization, you'll leave."

For so long, I'd been far away and safe. But, I was deeply engaged with what was happening there, if only in my own heart. I was not committed to Lawrence Academy as a school, nor to the culture or the region that had borne it. But, I was committed to something. It was time to name the nature of my commitment - to reconcile the tensions growing inside me.

"Only when you believe your actions matter, and care deeply, will you consider speaking up."

Speaking up means owning the risk that we will piss people off. We must be willing. We must know the conviction of our actions as necessary for the betterment of the world. At times, we must piss people off, just to protect our own dignity and rights. That alone is a worthy cause. Other times, we will have to piss people off to protect whole groups of vulnerable people.

Hatmaker also says, "If we are waiting on systems to overturn themselves, we're just gonna go to the grave in an unjust world. So, this work is ours to do."

No one else was going to do this. Steve Hahn and others' choices had wreaked havoc on my life, endangered many, and disenchanted so many others. My body would not tolerate it. Life would not tolerate it any longer. It was time.

Grant continues, "Fundamentally, these choices are based on feelings of control and commitment. Do you believe you can affect change, and do you care enough to try?"

I cared, and I was going to do more than try.

Already On My Way

"What drives you as an aspiration is to
'find strength in the discovery of what is true.'
And I think what you're describing is,
however hard the truth is,
it does complete us."

— Krista Tippet, speaking of Isabel Wilkerson

As I drove, my body was pulsing with a drive, and a rage, that fueled me to the point I felt I was nearly flying. It was my eighth trip across the country, and it had never felt like this. I would know this feeling many times.

I drove and drove and cleared my head. I was energized and focused by the time I got past the Rockies and on into the plains, I started to compose. That little voice recorder was the ideal tool to capture my message. I grasped it in one hand, watching the changing wintery landscapes of the country all around me. I would record by day and transcribe by evening.

I remember consciously deciding to leave out any descriptions of the stalking behavior in the speech - because I didn't want to scare the kids. To me, that has always been the most frightening aspect of what happened at Lawrence Academy.

Somewhere in the middle of the country, I stopped at a payphone to call my partner at home in California. He told me that Steve Hahn had called. "Oh, yeah?!" I exclaimed, with my pissed-off, defiant tone. "He said he wanted to talk about content.". I laughed! Well, he can go to hell, I thought. "What did you tell him?". My partner replied, "I said you were already on your way!" We both laughed.

Then, for the last third of the country, I was fueled not only by the urgency of the truth - but the anticipated fight of defending my First Amendment rights. He can't tell me what to say! There is no editing here. It's fucking show time. I was just a day or two away from Massachusetts when I called home to California again. My partner told me, "They sent a letter. Do you want me to open it?". "Yes!" He read and got to the line, informing me that they let Pete Regis go. He was released on "permanent long-term disability", it read.

I didn't think to question the terms of his removal at the time, because, well, I had finally done it! He was gone, and kids would be safer now. That's what it took. Their knowing I was on my way, and they could not reach me to control what I would say - that's what got a documented child-molester removed from campus.

It's fucking tragic when you think about it. The right decision was so obvious, and yet, it took me all of seven years to achieve what should have taken Steve Hahn five difficult minutes.

I would learn many years later, in 2018, that Steve Hahn had been telling his colleagues that he had "no idea why I was coming" and that I was "unstable". Talk about your sloppy defamation efforts. On a 23-year-old. My goodness.

~ ~ ~

On December 9, 2001, I pulled my truck into a motel parking lot in western New York and got myself a room. It was almost my 24th birthday. I laid all my notes out on the floor and stepped into the shower. I was speaking at Lawrence Academy the next day. I felt rattled by anticipation, but then so relieved to be in a hot shower. The ending of the speech suddenly came to me, "...because there's infinite power and freedom in having nothing to hide".

I stepped out, scratched these words down on paper, and cried in long, joyous release. After all I've been through, hearing my voice and the power of these words finally releases the tears to flowing. When I crumple into crying there, it feels triumphant.

I know it will be ok. Better yet, it's going to be a whole new kind of ok; it's all going to be renewed in health. The darkness of their silencing and secrecy is about to end. I can feel a new day bursting forth from within me, like the light of truth refusing to be contained by darkness - in a body, in a school, or a society - any longer. It is coming. I am happily floored by the power of it moving through me - literally bringing me to my knees.

The next day, my driving is calm, clear, and focused. I arrive right on time to my 2:00 speech. All three hundred-plus students, faculty, and staff are gathered inside that auditorium. It's just me steering the Toyota with the California plates into a spot behind the back-stage entrance. I've decided I am not giving any one of them the chance to intercept me. No one to urge me toward some watered-down message. I know these men. I know these tall, white colonial buildings. I can use that back door at ground level near the art studio and walk right onto stage left.

It's bitter cold, as it always is in Massachusetts in December. My heart is thumping, but my sight is luminous as I step out of the car. Mini-cassette recorder in hand. I inhale a chest-full of dry, cold New England air and see the steam of my breath as I step determinedly toward that doorway. It's unlocked, *success!* I breathe in again, remembering the power and significance of what I am about to do. I pull the door open toward me and hear a full auditorium of young and old voices anxiously murmuring in anticipation. I step inside . . .

~ ~ ~

Steve Hahn approaches me nervously when he sees me enter and move right toward the podium. He starts in on his prepared last-ditch effort, but I interrupt and say, "Look, I am only here to tell the truth - and I'm going to be kind.". There was nothing more he could do. How could he have possibly thought I would be loyal to his comfort and secrecy, after all of this? After they'd sent me away, after years and years of my pleading for right action.

Achillea's heel, indeed.

Now, if you are enjoying the audiobook, you can hear for yourself just how very "stable" I was on stage. I was calm. I was focused, and I was steady.

Steve approached the microphone and said, so very simply, "This is Vanessa Fadjo, and she graduated from Lawrence in 1996.". That was it. He backed away and slipped off stage.

I had never felt so entirely alone and so connected to something larger in my life. It was like walking into surgery, and knowing my partner and dear companion would be right there beside me. Or like sleeping in my car in the west Texas plains. I was loved and supported, yet I still had to do the hard part all on my own. Luckily, I had healed from surgery quickly. So I could stand solid on my own feet that day and not be moved.

I knew Sybil was somewhere in that big, anxious crowd. I imagined a few others who knew and loved me scattered among the seats. But, I couldn't see anything with the lights already hot-bright and glaring into my eyes on stage. I assumed the post, and Steve Hahn walked away.

Then, the auditorium was completely silent in anticipation. I laid the mini-cassette recorder on the podium, pushed Record, and began.

The Speech
December 10, 2001
Groton, Massachusetts

"Hello. Ok, so he gave the basics. My name is Vanessa and I graduated from Lawrence in '96. I guess that's all you've been told about why I'm here… I won't do that (fumble with the microphone). So, I'm here for a couple of reasons. And the first is that I have a story. And I have some insights about that story. And I have some words of guidance to offer you. Most of all, I'm here to break an unspoken pact between me and Lawrence Academy to keep a secret. I hadn't planned on saying this, but I understand some people might get upset. But, like I've told Steve, I'm only here to tell the truth - and I'm gonna be kind.

So, I came to Lawrence as a freshman in '93 from Catholic grade school. It was a school of mostly girls, and nuns and uniforms. I was happy to be here (I laugh a bit).

So, at the end of my freshman year, I was molested by Pete Regis, the groundskeeper."

— the whole place fell even another level of silent —

The first time, you know, it was subtle, and I think I just had a sense of shock and disbelief. 'This guy's my buddy - I tell him about my life and he teaches me about cars and... I mean, I was so inexperienced that I didn't even know how to recognize sexual abuse.

And so then, my fre- my sophomore year, a lot of events started unfolding really fast in a short period of time. I had had another experience with Pete - and this time I knew it was wrong because afterwards, he told me not to say anything because somebody might get the wrong idea. Soon after that, I told my boyfriend at the time, and of course, he was really upset. Soon after that, one of my best friends came to me and said Pete had done similar things to her.

Now, it was bad enough that it happened to me, but when I knew it had happened to somebody that I loved, we knew we had to do something. So, we met one day under this tree and wrote about all our feelings about what had happened. And when we were done, we shared it. And I had written mine in the first person, as if I was speaking to Pete. So, after that, we decided that we would go down and I would read that to Pete, what I had written.

And that was a pretty scary situation. We had no idea how he would react. My boyfriend skipped baseball practice and waited outside with his bat (laughter from the audience). My friend and I, ya, know, forged in there - and freaky as that was we knew the two of us together were stronger than Pete and what he had done.

I remember how bad my hands were shaking, ya know, as I held that little piece of paper that I never intended to share with him. And luckily for us, he hung his head and he nodded and agreed with everything we said.

After that, I learned that a woman who was working locally downtown... she had to be at least my age now at the time, had told me she was so glad that we did that because the same thing had happened to her years and years ago.

And I was blow away - just thinking about that... I mean, how many women did this happen to and for how long has he got... ya know, has this gone on.

So next, my friend and I - well, after we, uh, we had gone in and spoken to him we took the three of us, ya know, huddled together, took the little piece of paper and burned it, thinking that would mark the end of it. But, I never realized how things would play out. And I never thought that Pete would be employed here for another seven years.

Next, we got, my friend and I both, got letter from Steve Hahn in our mailboxes asking us to come and talk to him. We got there and it wasn't just Steve Hahn but Denny Blodgett, and the old dean Maura Delaney and someone from the Department of Social Services. Personally, I felt tricked. I mean, I would have liked more comfort and notice. But we sat there and gave details about what happened to these faculty and a stranger from a government office. My parents were never informed about what happened. And I think at the time, I bought into the shame of it.

And I'd had that really good martyr training in Catholic school about, ya know, I can just take the pain on myself and not have to hurt anybody else, and... But I look back and I denied myself support that I needed and I denied my family the chance to help me. And there's nothing honorable about looking past what you need.

So, after the uh, after the meeting - and that was pretty much the last outreach done by the school. My feeling was that the situation was very hush hush. And it was the dirty little secret. I asked what happen about this and I was told that Pete was going to be placed on a kind of suspension contract. That if he had interaction with students again, he would have to go.

So, from this I took that, well, two known times wasn't bad enough. And that the school was willing to take the risk with all of your safety, to keep him employed, for reasons I still don't understand. It was like, I knew it was wrong, but at the time I felt powerless. Ya know, I had always been taught to behold the glory of the 200 year old institution that is Lawrence Academy. I didn't think I could do anything about it.

So, soon, the year was ending, and I find mysteriously there's no money available for me to come back. And I hadn't been a great student. I wasn't making great grades - I had my share of level 2 offenses. But I wasn't failing and I wasn't on academic probation or suspension contract. I had done nothing to get myself removed from the school. So, I felt like I was being punished about being abused by one of their own.

A part of me was relieved to just be out of the whole mess. Ya know, I didn't know if I wanted to be a part of a place that could let something like this happen. But, on the other hand, I was heartbroken. I mean, this was the first place I had found the freedom to explore things that interested me. I created art and my opinion in English class mattered and I had found my love for modern dance. I had gone to Arizona with the school and discovered my traveling spirit. Ya know, and all of my friends were here and I loved them and they're still some of the best friends I've ever had.

So, I left Lawrence Academy and spent my junior year at public school in Acton. I would get the news that, yeah, Pete was still employed. As my senior year rolled around, it was really important to my parents that I graduate from a good name school. So they bargained with the school and pleaded for me to be let back in - and when I look back I think, what did I do?

So, under certain conditions, I was allowed to return to Lawrence Academy. And at this point I didn't care - because I had decided that, as soon as I was legally able to do it, I was gonna move to California. And I felt like I was just biding my time. So, I did return and I drudged through. I was really independent. I did some independent work and independent winterim. And barely, I graduated in '96.

(And then I moved to California within a month... I made it)

So, in '97, my sister was graduating from Lawrence. And I came back to Massachusetts and back to Lawrence to attend graduation. And the first face that I saw was Pete's. And I was Pissed. Because, the deal was supposed to be that he was gonna be kept behind the scenes. And I felt that, by what a prominent figure he was made, this deal wasn't taken seriously.

My friend who had been involved was also graduating that year. And then I had a realization that I haven't been able to let go of since. And it's that, anybody who was around when some noise was made is gone - and Pete's still here.

This upset me so much, thinking about it. That new kids were gonna come in and not know. So, this began my four and a half year correspondence with Steve Hahn. And all I've ever wanted was for him not to be here.

In my first letter to Steve, ya know, I was writing about how it's not fair and that I get the feeling that you know there's bad out there in the world, and you can see people suffering, but you don't know where it comes from exactly. And then we find a source of this corruption and fear - and we do what everybody else must be doing to explain this state - we look the other way.

At first, the response I got was that, 'Well, he's acted well, met them terms of the agreement and I don't see any reason to terminate his employment now.'. And he claimed that, at the time, they acted within the law.

And I've never had a big group of lawyers on My side, but I feel like I don't need that to know that it's wrong to knowingly employ a child molester at a place where groups of kids are going to come in every year and not know.

Later, it was that... and year after year, every time I returned to Massachusetts, and would stop into the office, I wrote letters. Later it was that Pete was gonna retire soon - and this gave me some hope, like ok, well maybe he just won't be there and they won't have to be in this situation.

So, I was here last spring and I had realized that, ya know, I know about it and I'm not really Doing anything. And so, I felt committed and I met with Steve in his office and we talked and I felt like, 'ya, he Really heard me and we're gonna get results'. And soon, the school year started and I hadn't heard from him. I was starting school. And... I got a publication in my mailbox out in California, I forget what it was called, but it said something about, ya know, there's something coming up where they're gonna ask alumni for their input about Lawrence Academy.

And I lost my patience here, because I thought, 'I've GOT shit to say'. So, we talked and I thought to come here and talk to you about sexual abuse.

Looking back over it, it seems the greater lesson is the abuse of power - but the two are connected. And so I've thought back on what I've learned over the last seven years… and I know that abuse happens both ways and that worse things happen. What I can share with you is what I've learned to be true from my experiences.

I believe that here you set the tone for your sexuality. Either you already have, or you're working on it, or you will in the next few years. And I think the tone of your sexuality will define whether or not you're gonna be likely to be abused. And it really strikes me that it comes down to your personal relationships, I mean the intimate relationships that you're already in, and the quality of those.

So, I really believe that it's important to know your body. Get all the information that you can about it. Don't be afraid of it. Trust it. I mean, it's hard to respect something that you don't know a lot about. And the more you learn, the more you will trust it.

And be aware of what feels comfortable to you. Ask yourself, 'Is this comfortable because it feels good and I like it… or, is this comfortable because it's familiar and it's what I'm used to?'. And you can work hard to imagine ideals, ya know, what a really balanced sexual relationship can feel like. And this is the kind of fantasizing that really pays off. It's like, I mean, really think of what that would mean to you in all the little details - and focus on that, and don't lose sight of it and don't settle for anything less.

I've noticed there's an idea that men are sexual and women are sexualized. And women are taught this, that ya know, you become the object of fulfilling a man's desire. But it's not true - women are equally as sexual as men are. And you just need to discover that for yourself.

Ya know and if something happens, and you feel like you've been wronged - Get Mad. Ya know, you're taught to be nice. And nice is dangerous. And the satisfaction of being true to yourself is gonna be a lot greater than the satisfaction of having been nice.

And for women, it seems like it comes down to this issue of rationing out. Like what am I going to give - here, and here, and here... but you can turn that around and think, ya know, what do I want to take and what do I Want from this situation - here and here. And you've just got to work on keeping it balanced.

As women, you can refine your intuition on views about you and your body. You can pay attention to comments and take them seriously... because these are clues into the attitudes about you and your body. And you can learn to avoid the ones that you know would play out in ways that wouldn't make you happy.

And as men, you can refine your views on women. You can see them as equally sexual. And in a way, this relieves a burden, because you can encourage your girlfriends and lovers to take initiative as often as you do - and really be equal with you. And you can... and you can empower the women that you're with.

And for both sexes, I think it's important to really say what you like and don't like. And it's always Ok to stop and say, 'Hey, ya know, I don't like this - let's do this.' Knowing what you want, and knowing what you will and will not take is part of how you define who you are. And it's an attractive trait.

And sexuality is a beautiful thing. Ya know, it's like any form of expression, you just need to be aware of what you're saying about yourself through how you're expressing yourself. And say things that you would be proud of.

And when I think back, and think what really would have helped me to hear, at that time, going through what I was going through... would have been to never view any sexual encounter, any person, ya know, institution, place, anything as greater than your self. I really wish I'd had the conviction seven years ago to say, 'This situation is wrong and I will not stand for anything less than this."And I hope that, by me telling you this story, you can learn to improve your own reaction time.

And if you see an injustice, call it and as fast as you can. Mine is just a small story in a bigger picture of stories that happen like this all the time. It's important to you for a few reasons. One, obviously is that sexuality is gonna always be a part of your life, no matter how it manifests. And, also just in terms of the world we're living in. With the advance of technology, there's a dehumanizing trend, and we're getting away from things that involve one-on-one human interaction.

And a lot of you are gonna go on to bigger name schools and work for even bigger businesses and corporations. And... groups like these are nothing if they're not made up of caring individual people. And their purpose in society at large is nothing if it doesn't meet the needs of individual people...if it doesn't honor what is human in each and every member of society.

And in that gap, where human connection once was, there's gonna be a lot of room for discrepancy of truth and crimes carried out. As I've seen more of the world and the way it works, I see things and they remind me of this story. When I've told it to people in California, I've heard amazingly similar stories. Where, uh, a girl told me that she went to a private school and was abused by one of the faculty members. She did tell her parents and they took her out of the school. Years later, she finds out the man who abused her had been promoted to administration and that they told the school that she was kicked out.

And there might be things in your life that remind you of this story. And... I encourage you to call an injustice as soon as you see it, not just against you but against somebody else. Martin Luther King, Jr. said that, "An injustice anywhere is a threat to justice everywhere.", and I really believe that.

In terms of the story... the most recent reason I got that Pete was still employed was that he had compelling health reasons that required insurance which he got from working here. So right before I got in the car to come out here, I got a letter and he informed me that Pete is no longer on campus. He's on permanent long-term disability. And I'm thrilled with this.

This means that Pete doesn't have to suffer physically for what he did, but it also means that you don't have to come back knowing there's a child molester on campus.

Now, I'm not here to turn you against Steve Hahn. I mean, for all the ways I would have liked things to go and any upset I have, he always sat down and listened to what I had to say. And I didn't know until recently the hierarchy of positions here, I mean, I think they're called regents (?), that are Steve Hahn's bosses, that he has to answer to. And, he's given me... and I know, and I see it, the side of Steve who really wants to do right by this situation. And he's given me the chance to be here and tell you. And I'm really grateful for that.

And I'm definitely not here to turn you against your school. This is a wonderful place, made of wonderful people and it offers... wonderful things (laugh). But I urge you to beware the institution that makes you feel small. Ya know, if there's something to be lost in your having a voice - don't trust it until you can question its objectives.

I have my theories on why... and I think I've said enough, so I'll leave them out. And they've all been... denied. I still don't know why. But I do know that this is a story in the past tense. This here today marks the end of the story. And I'm content because I know that should an injustice be brought to their attention, the school will handle the situation much more honorably and more thoroughly.

But it's gonna be up to you to bring it to their attention. Whether it's an injustice in your personal life and you need to bring it up to someone, to one person's attention, or here, or any place that you go. I encourage you to speak your own truth. No matter who you're speaking it to, and no matter what you're speaking it up against - because there's infinite power and freedom in having nothing to hide.

Thanks."

Waves of Reckoning

The applause lasted so long; the audience simply wouldn't let Steve Hahn speak. Each time he approached the podium, it would start up again, interrupting his gait and causing him to stumble backwards. He and I had agreed that he could speak after me. But, everything he said came out in muffled tones, like someone reaching for air while underwater. He was drowning in the truth of the situation and grasping for the old denial and justifications again. When really, he should have been reaching for the stronger grip on acknowledgment and apology.

He blundered a while. Then, faculty and staff lined up to shake my hand. My brother's girlfriend later pointed out that this was a political move. After what I'd revealed, each one wanted to be seen as standing on the right side of this. So, they lined up for whatever internal motivators, and I regarded them anew, as a 23-year-old woman, who had seen far more of the world at this point.

Sybil and I triumphantly hopped in my Toyota truck with California plates and drove the old loops around rural Groton. She was as energized as I've ever seen her. Generally, this woman is sturdy and subdued as a bull. So, it was always especially fun to see her animated and overflowing. "I wanted to stand up and scream, 'I was the friend!'". We reveled in the triumph together, just as we'd shared in the hardship and the pain. These are the ones we most need to celebrate with, after all.

~ ~ ~

Just weeks later, on January 6, 2002, The Boston Globe released their seismic Spotlight investigation into child abuse cover-ups in the Catholic Church. The headline read, *"Church allowed abuse by priest for years: Aware of Geoghan record, they still shuttled him from parish to parish."*[1]. The choice to knowingly shelter and protect these abusive men in power had finally grown intolerable in the collective consciousness. A wave of outrage erupted throughout the region.

I had no idea, at the time, that these waves were cresting simultaneously around New England.

The 2015 movie, *Spotlight,* directed by Tom McCarthy with co-writer Josh Singer, portrays the systemic silencing and institutional abuse by the Catholic Church. It tells the story of the challenge the investigative reporting team faced in breaking a stubborn silence. Most remarkable to me is the depiction of new Editor Marty Baron, and his role in elevating this story in Boston. He'd been brought in from Florida when The New York Times purchased the Globe in 1993.

He came from an entirely different region, and he was also Jewish: outside of Boston and outside of Catholicism. The "outsider" perspective was what allowed him to see that these stories - which had been slowly surfacing for years - actually were a big deal.

I've often thought, by removing me, Lawrence Academy officials gave me everything I needed to see them clearly and keep speaking the truth of the situation. I had become the outsider. They'd removed my belonging, and I had given myself the vast distance of seeing so much more beyond them. My perspective was instantly more expansive. Now, it was time to share that insight back in the place where young people were still unknowingly endangered.

---

[1] Globe staff, January 6, 2002, https://www.bostonglobe.com/news/special-reports/2002/01/06/church-allowed-abuse-priest-for-years/cSHfGkTIrAT25qKGvBuDNM/story.html

~ ~ ~

Before traveling east, I had the foresight to give my family a bit of notice, to let them know I'd be coming back to blow up that facade. I called my father first. As a big fish in a small pond, he knew a lot of people. His dental practice was in the center of town, and he talked openly about his life with his patients. I figured I would let him know before he heard about it from one of them. On the phone, he feigned upset and surprise. I also remember him commenting on my "still being upset about this" in a dismissive tone.

Fortunately, I became less and less tolerant of bullshit excuses, and more and more accepting of my own rightful anger over the years. I recognize now, in both the language of my speech and in my father's reaction, that a lack of accountability in men was condoned. At the same time, self-protective emotion in women was condemned in that time and place.

Of course, my father had never addressed the situation with me at the time. So, I believed this would all be news to him. His response was confusing, in the intentional way I have come to identify when people with something to hide say odd things that don't line up. I never knew about those phone calls from Steve Hahn to my father seven years earlier. I still don't know what kind of subtle blame, coercion, or lack-of-accountability was delivered by his voice over the unrecorded lines.

Amidst the confusion and obfuscation of my phone call back east, my father said he would be there. He was. My younger brother, Cameron, joined him in the auditorium. Cameron told me later that they had sat behind Katie Regis, Pete's wife (or soon-to-be-ex-wife, at that point), and how uncomfortable that was for him. My brother approached the stage afterward, like so many. When it was his turn to speak to me, he cried. "It's just so upsetting," he sniffed. That was the appropriate, humane response.

I'd told my sister before I traveled east too. She then got on the phone to the Lowell Sun while at my mother's photography studio in Chelmsford. My sister, Adrienne, recounted later how our mother walked into the room while she was speaking to a reporter. Realizing what was happening, my mother interrupted her by nearly screaming, *"Adrienne, what are you doing? Hang up the phone! How could you do that to Lawrence Academy?"*

I know. Whatever you're thinking, every one of those thoughts is valid.

~ ~ ~

In the Spotlight movie, reporter Matt Carroll visits the mother of one of the children who had been abused by a priest. The mother tells him, "There was a lot of pressure to keep quiet.". "From the church?" he asks. "Yeah, from the church," she confirms, and then continues, "But not just the church... from my friends, from the other parishioners".

During an interview with Globe reporter Sacha Pfeiffer, a man who'd endured abuse by a priest says, "The Bishop came over to the house. He said nothing like this had ever happened before and asked us not to press charges". She asks, "And what did your mother do?". He says, "My mother?" in an incredulous tone. "She put out frickin cookies.".

Remember, a compromised sense of survival tainted my parents' perceived position in that social stratosphere. They had been susceptible to any overt or covert messages that they were less-than and needed to stay in line. It is tragic. Yet, I imagine they felt threatened by my doing this; my mother alarmed by my sister's attempt to amplify what I was doing. Even if thwarted, it was a small gesture of solidarity on my sister's part, and I acknowledge that here.

It is a powerful statement on the culture of a place when it creates a gulf between parent and child, and a dividing line within families, over which a side must be chosen.

~ ~ ~

Steve Hahn resigned abruptly from the position of headmaster the following year. He left without a word of acknowledgment on the issue. I later learned, not one word was ever spoken to the student body following my speech. A former student who had been present in the auditorium told me years later, "It was so surreal.". He wrote to me about how unforgettable it was, seeing me tell that story, and how bizarre it was to then have the adults say absolutely nothing in response.

Not a word about Steve Hahn's choice to keep Pete Regis on staff showed up in public statements, either. It was all praise. Like the creation of Columbus Day, in the wake of his unthinkable brutality. Where does celebrating cruelty end and applauding silence over cruelty begin? What you cover for, what you stay silent for, and what you stand for soon all flows into the same thing. When the faculty approached me on stage, many had said, "I had no idea this was going on.". Some did. There may have been some in that line who wanted to shake my hand, only to be seen as standing on the right side of this issue. They could celebrate my success at 23, but not risk their jobs to protect me at 16. I know, in retrospect, contradictions abounded in that line, too.

Belonging - A Home in One's Heart

"You only are free when you realize
you belong no place
— you belong every place —
no place at all."

— Maya Angelou

My most important task was now complete. Or, it is more accurate to say, I accomplished the most significant step I could imagine at that point. So many times on this journey, I have arrived at new breakthrough places to think, "Ok, now it is done.". Only, the scope of what I needed to address widened with each new level. Now I see it through the physics of microcosm and macro. The reach of a social issue pans outward - one abusive man, one complicit administration, one ideology - until some furthest point when it breaks through to the deeply internal. The work then exists in one conscience, one life's decisions, one moment's motivations uncovered and examined - One heart.

I know I am not the first to be punished and sent away for speaking a truth that threatened an existing power structure. I could trace the long lineage of souls who risked position or belonging to honor what they knew was right. I would be humbled to count myself among them. Here, I want to give a moment to the rewards that come after taking the risk.

So, what is belonging? I consider belonging as devotion, an anchor, and a root. I feel in my bones the idea that we belong to certain lands and not the other way around. I have found sacred places on both sides of this country, nearly symmetrical mirrors of one another in wild nature, where I feel most at home. The relationships are ongoing, as I watch them change or stay the same, while I change and stay the same. I long for them periodically, to re-experience our mutual knowing, the way I long for spring after winter. Yet, for me, true belonging is a sacred place within myself. The reward of risking that kind of speaking is the discovery of this very Home.

When we value our true selves, more than a status quo, we begin to come home. Our integrity and our connections can co-exist and evolve together. Love is the place where both are possible. I have also learned, those who silence their internal dissent will criticize those who speak up for their rights, needs, or feelings. Beware of those who retaliate against an assertion of these truths, no matter what the realm. Any expectation of mutual self-betrayal is a contract for failure. Integrity is the prevention and the remedy.

Ultimately, and this is where true power lies: no one can cast you out of the home in your heart.

In my professional life as an adult, I've had the opportunity to ask many people what integrity means to them. Some of the best answers included:

- Consistency of thought, feeling, word, and action in line with one's highest values
- Speaking up when something is off, instead of getting all blocked up inside about it
- Unwillingness to compromise on your values, willingness to sacrifice for your values

Of course, these are all highly personal. What I know for myself is this: Integrity was my first experience of freedom in belonging. Integrity, for me, is a home.

There are so many levels of Home I am yet to experience . . .

From "Belonging: Remembering Ourselves Home" by Toko-pa Turner: "There is a pivotal juncture in every Heroine's Journey when she stands alone. She is led by the depth of her convictions to take a stand, to name the unaddressed, to call out of hiding the secret malaise in her community. She arrives at a standpoint not without doubts, but in spite of them. And sometimes, there is a hefty price to pay, like being the target of criticism, or worse, rejection from the group which is at odds with her truth.

"The willingness to rebel from the expected norms, roles, and silent contracts of establishment comes out of knowing that one cannot afford to build resentment. Resentment, which comes from the decision to go against one's truth, embitters the self. It somaticizes in the body and takes on the burden of pain as if it were ours alone. The whistleblower, on the other hand, reveals a shared complicity. It says, "I expect more from myself and from you." And in that stance the pain becomes, in a sense, communal."

When it comes to healing, we have to feel it, even the pain, and then deal with it. Sometimes, that itself is a journey.

Major Blessing - Chosen Coping Strategy

"I'm right there, swimming the river of hardships
but I know how to swim."

— Jack Kerouac

I have often been aware that I've been blessed to make it to this point because of my chosen coping strategy. By chance, I felt compelled to manage my trauma by driving across the country twelve times over a decade, which had its gifts. It was joyful and cathartic. Most of all, it was effective enough to protect me until I was ready to integrate where I'd been with where I needed to be.

I also smoked cigarettes for a different decade (ages 15-25). I don't recommend this to anyone. Smoking had its place in my coping strategies along the way. I am fortunate to be so physically healthy today. Whether it has contributed to diseases or not, I will not know for sure. Here's what I do know: Lungs want to heal, the way the soul wants to heal, and all healing only asks for our cooperation.

The road as a coping strategy cost me relatively little, considering all it gave. My recovery simply took time. My education and career advancement have followed a very different trajectory as a result.

It took me twelve years to earn my Bachelor's Degree, which I did entirely with my own money, and very much on my own terms. By the time that paper came in the mail, I had attended all of six colleges: three junior colleges, two state universities, and one adult-oriented interdisciplinary college in San Francisco. But, I stuck with it. I always went part-time, doing landscaping or waitressing work to pay my rent, bills, and tuition. It was the first time "education" meant something meaningful to me personally, and fed my purpose in the world.

Along the way to that Bachelor's Degree, I would face a number of real challenges...

~ ~ ~

If not for the road, and my ability to move freely for years with it, I could have had a different fate.

I want to take a moment to give a nod to the co-journeyers on the path to healing who resorted to drugs, alcohol, meaningless sex, or self-harm. I do get it. I extend a heartfelt empathy to those who survived at greater expense, and to the loved ones of those who barely survived, and those who did not. I acknowledge humbly that so many got in too deep and couldn't find their way back out. I feel the tragedy of that acutely. Some even chose to end the life they were given because the pain was too great.

A moment of silence for those who were lost to the impacts and their attempts to get through.

Every life has its grace and its glory.

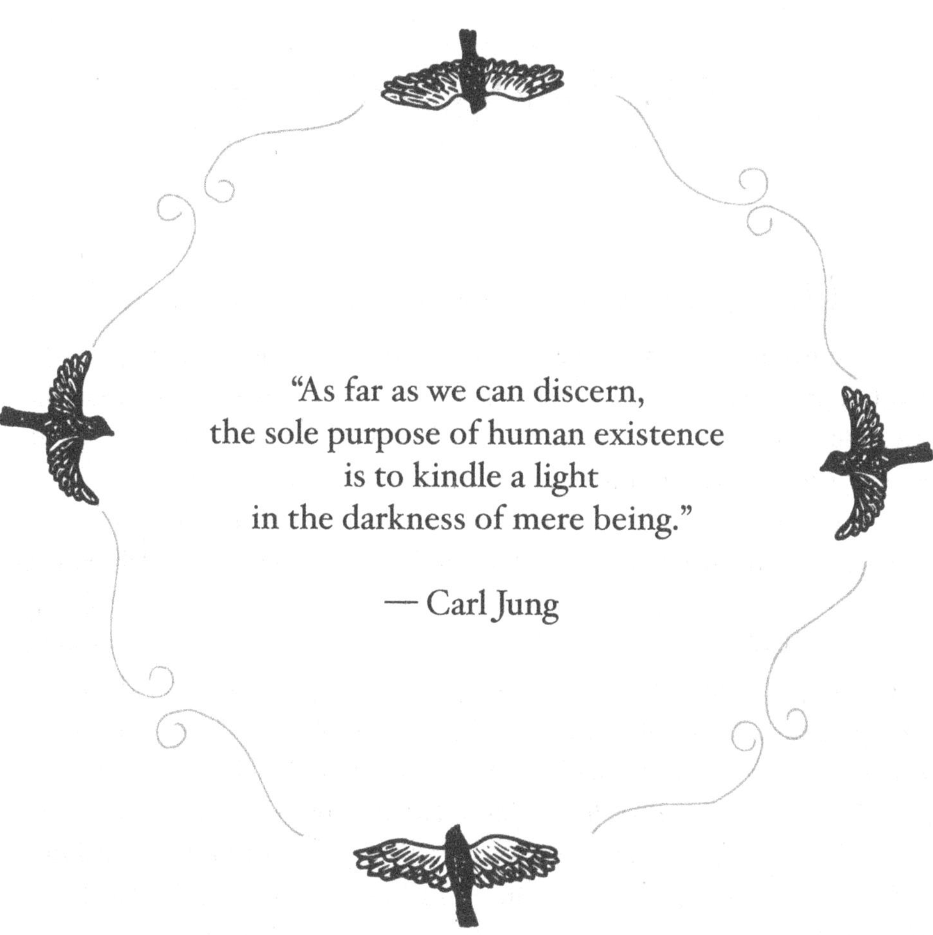

"As far as we can discern,
the sole purpose of human existence
is to kindle a light
in the darkness of mere being."

— Carl Jung

The Body Speaks - 2005

Healing trauma means releasing increasing amounts of stored pain, as our bodies and souls are ready to process it. There is an undulating rhythm that brings us to an edge of intensity and then recedes. We gather strength, integrate what was released, rest, and then are washed toward a new edge of growth, whether we are consciously ready or not.

I lived in Northern California for four years in total. I had an intimacy with the place, and I was known there. Yet, an ungrounded agitation still urged me on. In my mid-twenties, I traveled up into the northwest and over the Canadian border to British Columbia. There, I stayed with a soulful family on Salt Spring Island who gave me something I'd longed for since leaving home: a model of a way of life I respected. We even knew similar people in Northern California. They were farmers and body-workers, raising their daughter on ten acres, living slowly, and fully present with one another.

When they were traveling to Cuba a few years later, they invited me to stay on their farm as a retreat. Since I had a month to myself, I decided to take another big step in healing and give up cigarettes. I figured if I was going to be cranky and in withdrawal, it would just be me, the chickens, the dogs, and the sheep. I could do this.

I carefully emptied packaged cigarettes onto newspaper, mixed the tobacco with an herbal blend, and filled them back up. It was a decreasing-tobacco and increasing-herbal blend plan. The movement of my hands was a meditative way to spend quiet evenings by the fire with their border collies. I read a book about quitting smoking over those weeks and endured a few more humbling nights of jumpiness and nightmares. The old sensations arose again for release. It was a gift to do it in a place where I felt safe, by a strong association with loving friends.

I cleansed my system slowly. I cut my long hair short. I welcomed my friends home from their travels and headed home to Northern California. I worked as a preschool substitute teacher, and I remember a few of my young students didn't recognize me. One five-year-old girl I'd cared for intermittently for years looked up at me and said, "You look vaguely familiar..." It kind of broke my heart.

But, I did feel changed. I had outgrown many things. Soon, I was ready to relocate again. I'd saved some money and decided to put all of my education in ecology and environmental resource engineering into action on a piece of land in Junction City, Oregon. It was five acres in the floodplain between Eugene and Corvallis, Oregon, with Bear Creek meandering through the oaks and cottonwoods.

~ ~ ~

Living on that land was my first experience of being at home and creating a meaningful life, with the intention to stay.

I was still working away at my Bachelor's Degree and attending the University of Oregon part-time. Sure, folks were starting to look young to me at 27. This school was by far the most populous and elaborate University I'd attended yet. But, I adored my classes. Sociology was a great fit for me, especially where I could find the intersection with gender and the natural world.

I waitressed part-time in Eugene with a fine group of people who made their small Greek & Indian Restaurant feel like a home. I would bike seven miles up the river trail to where I'd parked my truck, load up the bike, and drive seven more miles to my land in Junction City, Oregon. There, I would tend my ducks, chickens, sheep and dogs, and cat. Country life is a balm to me in a similar way that the road was, and I was finding new access points to soothing my soul that could support health. I was learning to play guitar and would spend hours in the back field, singing among the cottonwoods. It was a blissful time. I had good friends and a well-balanced life.

Then, about two years into my time on the land, I had an experience with a man that echoed the old stalking pain, the most profound trauma from my days at Lawrence Academy. There is a tragic way we play out our past wounds to understand them fully and finally heal. Releasing my coping mechanism of running away was necessary for a successful life. Yet, it was only in facing the pain again that the compulsion would start to change shape.

With that pain reactivated, my body responded in quick and certain terms: Growths. Large endometriomas on the top and bottom of my left ovary. I could barely go to work. Soon, it hurt to laugh, which seemed the cruelest of circumstances. I also knew, from a very young age, that motherhood was absolutely for me. Being able to have my own child was as innate to my nature as breathing was to my body. There was no question.

My urge to stay at my home in Oregon was so strong and reinforced by my life circumstances (I had a mortgage). I loved that land with a depth that has never left me. I still dream of it now, sixteen years later. I didn't have smoking as a crutch anymore. I was also no longer actively fighting for the protection of others (Pete Regis was finally off Lawrence Academy's campus).

So, it was all getting back to myself. Whether I felt ready or not, it was time to integrate every one of the pains.

~ ~ ~

In 2018, Johns Hopkins released a report, "One Year's Losses for Child Sexual Abuse in U.S. Top $9 Billion, Study Suggests"[2]. In it, the

2 Johns Hopkins Bloomberg School of Public Health, May 21, 2018, https://www.jhsph.edu/news/news-releases/2018/one-years-losses-for-child-sexual-abuse-in-us-top-9-billion.html

economic impact from 2015 from costs associated with health care, child welfare, special education, violence & crime, suicide and survivor productivity losses was calculated at $9.3 Billion. [U.S. families spent $144 Billion on private high school tuition that same year] Who is carrying the burden of those behaviors, and who is responsible?

I sat with a surgeon again at 27, in Oregon this time, and felt intolerant to everything she was saying. She spoke casually, in some aloof, almost powerless tone about the upcoming procedure. She said, "I'd hate to take your ovaries because you're so young". I instantly snapped back, "I won't let you take either of them". I left that clinic immediately.

While I'd struck gold with Madeline from Planned Parenthood of Eureka, California, and the wonderful team at the local hospital, I just kept striking out in Eugene, Oregon. The state healthcare system was far less-funded and for some reason, I met only under-qualified folks. My next attempt was with a female surgeon of about 50. She was overly-nice and indirect in her way of speaking with me. I'm east coast, after all. I want people to tell it to me straight.

I started losing trust as she spoke more and more of her father, who was also a surgeon. She started to imply that he would also attend, which confused me. I said, "But you would be the one doing the surgery, correct?". She said, "Oh, yes, of course. We just like working together."
I thought, sarcastically, *'Right, but it's not a social event, it's my body.'*
She was losing ground with me by the minute. Then, she said, "So, when we remove your ovary, I mean, the cysts..."

I cancelled my appointment that afternoon.

I had to have surgery. I was not able to function physically for stretches of time - which was especially hard while living alone in the country. State healthcare was not providing what I needed, so I started exploring all options to find medical help elsewhere. Poignantly, this meant I would eventually end up on the east coast. Everything began pointing to the fact that I would have to revisit my roots to achieve health now. I didn't want to go. But, my body had spoken, and all that was left now was to respond.

In part surrender, part tragedy, I started unwinding the beautiful life I'd created. Everything I had outrun finally caught up with me in another horrible stalking experience, and medical problems immediately followed.

I had to withdraw from classes at the University of Oregon, leaving a D grade on my college records, followed by a W for withdraw. I got tenants for my land and left my job for an indefinite period of time. Endometriosis brought everything to a halt, and I was packing my whole life into some artificial Hold button. I prepared to return to Massachusetts to have surgery in Boston.

~ ~ ~

Dr. Holly Harris, epidemiologist at the Hutch Cancer Research Center, authored a report calling the association between childhood abuse and endometriosis "particularly strong". The findings, released in the Journal of Human Reproduction in July 2018[3], cited a 79% higher risk of developing the condition in those who reported severe or chronic abuse.

Every time I sat in that opulent New England headmaster's office from 1994-2001 and Steve Hahn repeated, 'This isn't a big deal', it aggravated the old pain in a chronic way. According to Licensed Mental Health Counselor, Jenny TeGrotenhuis, "Invalidation is a form of relational trauma which, over time, harms the brain and nervous system.". I stand by the choice to continue returning despite the invalidation because the alternative carried its own pain (allowing the risk to incoming students). Yet, meeting that situation unchanged for so long meant an ongoing panic for me. Chronic injustice at the school became chronic pain in my body.

Dr. Holly Harris continues, "Both physical and sexual abuse were associated with endometriosis risk. And it's a strong association. There's also a dose-response, meaning the risk increases with increasing severity and type of abuse." When the condition flared up for me again in 2005 in Oregon, it

---

[3] Fred Hutchins Cancer Research Center, July 17, 2018, https://www.sciencedaily.com/releases/2018/07/180717125826.htm

brought all of my beautiful new life to a complete halt.

The Johns Hopkins report captures this well. "It affects quality of life, it causes loss of work.", said senior author Dr. Stacey Missmer of Harvard and Michigan State Universities. Once we see the correlation between child abuse and the real costs to our country, can we take these impacts seriously?

What I knew was the impacts of institutional abuse were now altering my life in every practical way. I packed my things into a spare room on the property, loaded up my cat and two dogs, and rented a trailer to pull behind my Toyota pick-up, across the country once again. As the days grew shorter and darker in late fall 2005, I began the slow crawl back to the original place of danger. With no other options and no possibility of escape, I threw my hopes into transforming it all into physical safety.

~ ~ ~

My friends stayed connected and loving as I went east again. I believed I would only be away for four months. The plan was surgery, recovery, and back to my life. But, I ended up staying in Massachusetts a full year. That journey east is foggy now, as things often are when your life falls apart, and you can't remember which terrible thing happened in what order. But, I do remember being in physical pain as I drove across the country, yet again, this time with a small tow-trailer of only the most essentials in my life. I had my two dogs and my cat with me in the truck. This amazes me as I think of it now: the whole caravan of us were traveling east in my least-thrilling, most heartbreaking journey back to my roots. My belly aching the whole time.

I remember the physical pain in my abdomen during a few stair-climbs to a motel room, with cat-in-crate, one giant breed Great Pyrenees on a leash, and a medium-sized Aussie mix on another. I had a surrender-moment, thinking, "This is all truly more than I can handle." And it wasn't the animals. It was hobbling back to my roots with these creatures I loved, my body breaking down from the inside. Of course, being able to get surgery when you need it always brings a humble gratitude. Crawling back to the place you ran away from ten years later in seeming defeat just sucked in ways I couldn't have imagined.

My return in 2006 was the first time I travelled east without the task of working to remove Pete Regis. It had been primary in every revisit to that point. I hadn't even been back east in over two years. Now, with my previous purpose gone, it was all dealing with the aftermath. Being so focused on protecting others had served as an adrenaline-override, where the real pain of my experience hadn't gotten space to air out yet. Who knew that caring for others was its own, secondary coping strategy? Now, I was surrounded by the space for it all to be released. It was all that was left around me.

I had arranged for housing at one of my favorite places in the world, Nagog Hill Farm, on the border of Acton and Littleton, Massachusetts. This was an ancient apple and peach orchard (it is said, the oldest in the country, planted by the natives in the 1600s) and a modern-day You-Pick Farm and commercial apple operation. It is home to Nagog Pond, the drinking supply for the town of Concord, and a protected wild area with trails up over the hills.

Charles Auger managed Nagog Hill and brought in seasonal laborers from Jamaica to work the orchards in the spring and summer. He and his wife lived in the main farmhouse at the corner. Since my surgery was scheduled for late fall, just after the apple harvest, I arranged to live in the workers' housing during my recovery. I figured I'd be quickly back to Oregon by the spring.

But, since this was a full-fledged, life-falling-apart experience, I learned that my housing had fallen through just a week before I was set to arrive. I couldn't make other arrangements that quickly, and still make it to my surgery on time. I had to focus on getting safely across the country. My tenants were already moving onto the property in Oregon, so I had to ride that momentum forward.

So, there I was, about to turn 28, settling into my father's basement with my two dogs and cat as I prepared for abdominal surgery. As someone who had highly valued my independence - both financial and personal - this was a devastating blow. I could surrender for a time to the necessary medical help my body needed. But then, my stay in Massachusetts became longer and longer. Soon, it morphed into a necessary, subconscious task of emotionally unpacking and repacking. I unpacked some of what I'd brought with me from my past, yet no longer needed. Then, I packed up other things I didn't want to leave behind.

I'd run away at 18, and now I was back, flat on my ass (as the east-coasters say) a decade later with nothing to do but look at it all.

~ ~ ~

The surgery was successful and they were able to save both of my ovaries. The masses (there were two) were large, dark, grey clouds on the ultrasound, blotting out the tiny sun of my left ovary. It was a maelstrom of pain in there. Given the task, of removing that much tissue and fluid from such a small space, I have to give respect to the man who did the surgery at Brigham & Women's Hospital in Boston. He was South American, which endeared me to him as I sensed a different kind of awareness in how he lived and viewed health. His presence was comforting.

Recovery took longer than I expected, and the negative melodrama of my father's current life situation was its own detriment to my health. My parents had finally divorced, and my dad had married his assistant soon after. That embarrasses me in ways I can't describe. Right about the time of my surgery, they, too, were divorcing. For many years prior, when I returned to New England, I would often feel consumed by my family (except my mother, her being absent), who were starving for a positive, female presence. They needed someone warm, protective, and loving. I would return to rest and replenish, and they would eat me alive. Of course, as one of the children, it was not my job to fill this role. But, they each tried to recruit me all the same.

If they were going to come to me, hungry for the same kind of nurturance they had in previous years, I was going to have to do something else. I couldn't recover while they fed off whatever strength I had left. I had energy enough to research apartments on craigslist, make phone calls, and visit places. My father, not a fan of animals or germs, was also growing impatient with our tenancy downstairs. He reached his breaking point on the dog situation one day and blew up. It was time to go.

This put me in an even more tragic position, as my income had stopped weeks prior. I had very little to float me, and I was starting to max out my credit cards. I have avoided debt like the plague, opting out of credit cards, until they were absolutely necessary financing my land at 26. When I began talking to credit unions in northern California, in hopes of soon buying land, a loan officer said to me, "Geez, I've seen people come down from the hills have more credit than you." Indeed, I had been under-the-radar in so many ways all of those years. My father's negative example of excess and debt taught me to be thrifty and to live well within my means.

The credit cards would be one of many concessions I would make over the years, to live fully in society again, at my own pacing and comfort level. So, having hit bottom in New England, I went looking for a place to stay while in my first home-region. I was able to find an off-season rental in the town of Newbury, on the New Hampshire coast. In the dark, emptiness of winter, the orange glow of the Seabrook Nuclear Power Plant radiated in the distance. It was not charming. Just miles from those beaches, I had walked the coastline at sunrise at 17, planning my escape. So, it was almost comforting and familiar in that way. But, this was November in New England, and the place was a ghost town with its own eerie sense of emptiness.

In some ways, if you go with the 'If you find yourself falling, dive' approach to transformation, it all kind of fit. This was the darkest, emptiest, most dreary place for me to wait out the winter of my eventual rebirth. Some deep, spiritual shifts were taking place after extracting the physical manifestation of all that pain. I was finally facing all I'd run away from:

the addiction of my parents,
the tendency toward betrayal,

elitist secrecy and silencing,
valuing image above reality,
the culture that produced and encouraged these kinds of priorities.

I'd had a ten-year respite from the close-up view. Then, I had to look at it straight-on and acknowledge every piece.

Soon, in my unthinking mode, my motions started proving resourceful. I was like a plant whose foliage had died. Slowly, subterranean roots were drawing in nutrients from further reaches of the soil by their own wisdom. I typed up a friendly letter and placed it in the mailbox of any home with a carriage house that looked livable. If they had space and would consider renting it to me with my animals, please drop me a line. I'd left a new message with Charles Auger, this time about the little converted chicken coop that sat on a small hill overlooking the pond. I noticed it seemed to sit empty. I told him to please let me know if anything opened up.

I was not running away as fast as I would have liked, that was for sure.

~ ~ ~

I fell into that depressive lull that comes when struggling against the changes only makes you tired, and the tides of life sweep you in... and out, in... and out. I was surviving. I am sure my whole system was resetting itself, but I was mostly silent as I moved through uninspiring days. I must say, it was from this place that I wrote my first full song and put it to music on the guitar. At least, I was starting to create from within the fertile darkness.

Then, one day as I drove Interstate 93, I got a call with a local 978 area code to my cell phone. Yes, I had finally adopted a cell phone at this point. I answered, and it was Charles Auger. He told me the woman writer who rented his little chicken coop had ended her lease and, 'Did I still want to live there?'

Dawn had broken on the horizon. I drove right away to Littleton, Massachusetts, and met him there on-site. The place was reverently quiet, surrounded by an enchanted landscape of water, trees, and softly rolling hills. The converted chicken coop was charming inside, with a functioning kitchen, a front room, a sleeping room, and a bathroom. Mr. Auger said, "It doesn't have running water, but you can pour buckets down the drains and it will work just fine.".

"That's ok!", I exclaimed. I would fill them in the nearby creek for the black and grey water systems, and go to a grocery store or to friends for drinking water.

Despite the extra work of "carry water", the place was cozy and warm. One wall was all windows that looked out over the most idyllic New England landscape I'd ever known. I was ecstatic.

We made an agreement for a very reasonable rent. He handed me the key and drove away. I stood at the door of my new home and cried in overwhelming relief. I was at home.

~ ~ ~

I stayed a full year in Massachusetts, to my utter surprise. By the time spring rolled around, a remarkable, yet ordinary thing happened. It was, of course, the spring of my ten year high school reunion. This struck me as entirely amusing, as it did Sybil, who was glad to be seeing more of me around New England again. Though she was a year younger, her brother had been in my grade, so she was very aware of the event. Did I want to go?

It was all so impromptu and spontaneous. I hopped on last-minute to join this small group of old friends at an event I wouldn't have even registered from my life on the west coast. Not something I would have traveled for, you can imagine. But hell, since I was there, I figured I could crash that party. I hadn't stepped foot on campus since the speech that brought exposure and change, and a wave of what else, I could only wonder.

I remember when faculty started recognizing me, five years after the speech, there was a noticeable fear and panic on their faces. I smirked a bit at this. "Oh, you've decided to join us?" a few asked. No, I hadn't signed up or paid for a ticket. For the very first time, it occurred to me, *'You know, they kind of owe me one. Of course, I'll take a lobster dinner on them'.*

It was part prank, part revelation - and just the insight I needed to set a new course of action.

My defiant delights all turned sour when I saw Steve Hahn there, wining and dining with the rest of them. Since he'd resigned right after the speech, he hadn't been headmaster for a good four years. Yet, there he was. What does it say of the school's standards that he was welcomed back with open arms? I last saw him in 2001, slumped in his chair in the auditorium as I revealed the truth he'd worked so hard to conceal for so long.

We talked, in that same absurd tension we always had - where I knew he was full of shit, and he knew I knew, and we laughed at pretending to talk above that truth all the same. He told me he was now headmaster at a different school, in New York state. This news hit me hard. How were people not caring about unethical behavior?! Though, it provided an important insight: it helped me realize the limits of the impact of that speech. I thought my arrival in 2001 would mean they would only make ethical choices from there on out. I thought Steve Hahn wouldn't be elevated to the status of leader ever again, given how he'd misused the role at Lawrence Academy of Groton, Massachusetts.

But, the taproot of denial runs deep - and the urge to make things seem ok even when they are not is the-air-they-breathe in elitist culture. It's what everyone always did without thinking. So, I now had my first glimpses into understanding, my work was not yet done.

Arrivals

After that major surgery in Boston, I moved regions again. I felt like an earthquake had torn through the beautiful life I'd made in Oregon, and it was only fragments when I returned. I didn't even return to settle. I stopped in for the business of tending my affairs and made my way very slowly into the northwest again. I had a new relationship, with a man I met right there in Concord, Massachusetts, where I was born. He and I traveled separately, and for different personal reasons, to the west coast. He, for the first time. Me, for the eleventh time, coast to coast, east to west again.

In 2007, I did another stint in California, living again in the San Francisco bay area. He lived nearby in Santa Cruz County. We had our separate but connected lives. It was funny, being back precisely ten years later. At 19, I'd lived in cooperative student housing in Berkeley. There, I met a man, and we bought one-way tickets to Hawaii - such a nineteen-year-old thing to do. After a decade of life and adventures, I got to see it all again with new, matured eyes.

This time, I stayed in a charming backyard cottage in Alameda, California. I rode the ferry over to San Francisco to attend classes at New College in the Mission district. I sold my land in Oregon, just three years after purchase when the market was favorable to me. With the return on my original investment, I was able to pay for school in full and finally wrap up that Bachelor's degree at 29 years old.

~ ~ ~

That fall, the man from the east coast and I traveled around the northwest with my Great Pyrenees dog. We were each untethered from our roots and yet to tie into anything lasting in a new home. So, we wandered together. I was even more like a seed dispersed on the wind now; I'd stopped voluntary contact with my mom at age 23, and then with my father at age 29. I wrote each one a letter, thanking them for everything I could think of, and sharing my reasons. I set healthy boundaries on any contact received from there on out.

It was odd in a way, having a companion on what had always been such a private mode, traveling where I felt drawn, and then setting up. I felt self-conscious, unsure as I was of the enduring value of living this way. I was aware that my twenties had not fit a mainstream experience. Yet, it was also wonderful to have a co-adventurer, to share joy, tenderness, and the excitement inside the unknown. It was a thrill to add wilderness backpacking to my way of knowing a new landscape.

We drove north to Washington together and crossed the Canadian border to visit my friends on Salt Spring Island. Then, we diverged in our respective trucks while I traveled alone to Montana, and he explored the gulf islands. We met back up in Bellingham, Washington, and discovered the town together. How sweet it was, to have a young man waiting, full of anticipation at the promise of creating a new life together. We chose a rental in late 2007 in Everson, Washington, and set up our first, stationary shared home.

~ ~ ~

He and I made one full, cross-country trip together - somewhat spontaneously - just a month later. While we'd met on the east coast, this time, we traveled west-to-east as a unified force. I finally met his family, and he met my siblings. We returned to Washington and a new time of discovery.

Then, in 2008, I gave birth to a child. My Gramma died just weeks later. I got to talk to her on the phone before she went. "Gramma, I had a girl.", I told her. In her tired, yet wise and loving voice, she brought a few words forth, "I know, honey, I saw the pictures... I don't think I'm gonna make it, Nessa".

She stayed with me long enough to see life regenerate and complete the circle of love she'd handed to me in her lifetime. My daughter, her first great-grandchild. Once, in my teens in Chelmsford, Gramma said to me, "I hope I get to make it to see you become a mom, Nessa. You'd be such a wonderful mother". This amazed me because I'd had the very same thought just days before. It was such a familiar magic, to hear her say the words out loud that I'd already carried within me. "I do too, Gramma.". We did.

My world shifted on a new axis, and I felt aligned with the person I was most meant to be. After so many departures, on so many levels, I was at home now more than I had ever been before. I had arrived.

Encounters

"Every year is a year of impact,
a month of change and a day of
new encounters.
It's all in the mind to make the impact,
see the change and conquer new
encounters."

- Kabelo Mabona

Major Blessing - My First Love

The encounters I had with Lawrence Academy groundskeeper, Pete Regis, all occurred before I had any practical experience of my own sexuality. I was so young and sheltered; my sexual development was unfolding on an entirely different path to those scary moments in Pete's shop.

It's important to be clear and admit honestly - the wound for me wasn't sexual. Sure, Pete had tried to distort sex and power to act out his disease. With some, I know the connection was tragically much clearer. He'd used deception and betrayal of trust to create unsafe situations for kids. Sexuality was the undertone of his predation, while the overtone was abuse of power.

It was the institutional abuse by Steve Hahn, and those who removed me instead of a child molester, that left the lasting impact.

Fortunately for me, the impacts of Pete's actions lingered for only a short while, until I found my connection to sexuality with my first love, Blake, in the seasons that followed. Since Blake had played a role in the confrontation, all of the recovery and the joyful discovery beyond was shared, as well. I was incredibly blessed.

Blake's smile was wide, bright, and radiant like the sun. He strode with a flowing mane of blond hair and a music in his gait. Sometimes, he'd even put that music to the harmonica as he walked. He would hike through the New England woods, singing loudly the contents of his soul, when no one could hear, relieved for the depths finding free expression at last. He was like

John Muir and Mick Jagger both, with a poet's soul and a brilliant mind.

We were naturally drawn to each other right away, the year he arrived. I was a sophomore, and he a new junior. He had an easy generosity and a hearth that glowed beneath a simple, New Hampshire-born kindness. For Valentine's Day that year, he hand-drew me a card and quoted Walt Whitman's poetry. With him, I felt safe and alive in ways I never had. He told me he fell in love with me one night, during a group adventure with friends, as I sang out in the dark of the passenger's front seat. I could feel that hearth reaching beyond his chest and inviting mine. Some magical alignment was forged.

We were each other's first love, and our connection became a doorway to new levels of love that expanded both of us.

To have my true introduction to love and sexuality shared with such a bright, brave, and honest man was an immense gift. I soon discovered that sexuality brought so much joy, satisfaction, and powerful healing connection. Knowing this, I felt all the more dumbfounded by the cultural secrecy around sex. It was absurd to me that those things had intersected at all. I thought,*'Who knew this was what they were keeping from me?!'* Then, I soon realized, "*This* is what Pete was trying to mess with?" No. Hell no.

As I grew, I recognized that sexuality itself, as a force in our North American culture, was vulnerable where it stood. Sex education had been entirely absent from my life, so to meet sex this way - after first navigating its dark shadowy-side - was a revelation. From where I'd grown back east, sex was cast aside as shameful, secretive, and somehow wrong. Souls were separated from bodies for generations. I'd heard stories on the west coast too, where kids were shown too much freedom around sexuality at the other extreme. This also didn't serve. People in America seemed to be vacillating at all sorts of unhelpful extremes - blindly trying to make sense of this aspect of being human.

It so clearly didn't have to be this way.

Sexuality was too sacred to be stranded there in the shadows. Who did this serve? Well, I knew of one person... What did that placement protect, really? So, that tumultuous journey from witnessing the cultural shadow of sex to experiencing the ecstatic light it offered awakened in me a fierce protectiveness of sexuality. No one was going to mess with this aspect of humanity, not if I could help it.

Blake also held a rare gift in creating courageous emotional intimacy with me. So, the emotional, physical, and spiritual aspects were always linked, and the vitality in each enhanced every other one. My true entry-point into sexuality was divinely placed. Those kinds of firsts cast a warm hue of color to our souls, that grows along with us, no matter how far apart our lives may take us.

Blake graduated at the end of the year I was sent away. So our time together was cut short too quickly. We'd talked about running away to California together, but that first year apart at different schools, me living out the extreme pain of retaliation and displacement, took its toll. Profound as any first love is, it is always coupled with inexperience. We didn't know how to manage a forced separation well. So, things became further disconnected for us as I grew withdrawn, disenchanted by all I'd seen, and so eager to leave the east coast.

~ ~ ~

There are so many ways we can leave one another.

Some people leave by getting lost in addiction. Some people stop feeling and dampen their own souls as a means of slow exit. Others collapse in shame. Even flying into a rage is a form of checking out, of leaving. I left the east coast physically in 1996 for my own, internal survival. Then, I left small towns and west coast regions entirely, over and over again, mostly because my capacity to stay and tolerate the old pain was so low.

I know humbly, and with a heavy heart, that I caused pain by all my leavings.

While our minds might understand that the person we love who leaves us is limited, and this causes separation, our hearts are not so easily convinced. Our hearts expand or contract in response to the real need for a human connection that will last. We can't know what will endure. It wasn't the people I was meeting on the west coast who I needed to leave. It was something in me that was still too rattled and overwhelmed to allow for a consistent, regular life.

Even with all of my limitations then, I definitely didn't want to leave Blake.

I often read how child abuse at the institutional level has ripple effects on a community. It was easy for me to believe in the early stages that my pain in being sent away was mine alone. Yet, here is homage to that truth. I see now, the way those closest are most buffeted about by the ripple of the boulder of corruption dropping into a young person's life. That child, and everything close to her, tipped off balance in concentric circles...

For the road of healing, the love between two people can be a profound source of steadying and connection. Blake and I held on while we could. I count my first love as a great blessing, as I always have and always will.

Definitions

cor·rup·tion | \ kə-ˈrəp-shən

1a
: dishonest or illegal behavior especially by powerful people (such as government officials or police officers) **:** DEPRAVITY
b
: inducement to wrong by improper or unlawful means (such as bribery)
the *corruption* of government officials
c
: a departure from the original or from what is pure or correct
the *corruption* of a text
the *corruption* of files

According to *Transparency International*,

Corruption is the abuse of entrusted power for private gain. It can be classified as grand, petty and political, depending on the amounts of money lost and the sector where it occurs.

Corruption corrodes the fabric of society. It undermines people's trust in political and economic systems, institutions and leaders. It can cost people their freedom, health, money – and sometimes their lives.

On the Whys & Recovery

People have asked me why I don't share sexual abuse details. So, let's go ahead and talk about the Whys.

We'd have to start by examining the word "victim". Consider that everyone, by the age of adulthood, has endured some kind of hurt or pain, often through someone close to them. So, is everyone a victim? I imagine a child walking into a nurse's office with a skinned knee and declaring, "I'm here because I'm a victim now.". It's overly simplistic and reductive to perceive ourselves this way. Even "survivor" is just a euphemism for an identity-based concept of one who has suffered and lived.

It is more accurate to say that we all have wounds. A "wound" is a point of negative impact, a tender place - emotionally, psychologically, sexually, spiritually, or interpersonally - that will need time and attention to repair. You can locate a wound, as separate from other places in the system that are still working optimally. These functioning places may need to go into overdrive to begin the healing process. But the wound exists in relative proportion to other points of strength.

There is an odd cultural phenomenon at play where we have confused experiences with identities. When so many advertise their successes and apparent 'perfections' online, there can be a strange flip-side: once someone reveals their suffering, people often place them into a lesser-than, spectacle category. Victim identity. We are so reluctant to own our wounds that we find relief when it can all be cast onto someone else who is "shown" as weak or damaged.

The first Why is because revealing private details evokes this kind of thinking. Like breaking the code of 'present-only-perfection' means it's now a free-for-all. I do not support this. Also, when we have only one of two undesirable categories to fall into: victim or perpetrator, everyone gets jumpy about their mistakes and their vulnerabilities both. We are not mature enough, collectively, to hold those and see clearly. Again, it becomes too polarized and loses shades of strength and meaning along the way.

Secondly, even when someone has endured a hardship, they still have a right to their dignity. On the other side of living through hardship is still a whole human being. You have suffered. I have suffered. People who suffer possess the very same rights as those who pretend to have not suffered. Everyone has the right to decide what they do with their personal information. I am affirming the rights of all people who have endured anything by my choice.

Third, people have a visceral response to graphic details - and this reaction is what lingers. I imagine many of you have encountered grim and shocking details of church or other private school abuse stories. Do you remember the context in which the events happened? *Probably not*. You (as a human) are only rattled by the physiological sensation of having read those details. Being disturbed is the main impact.

Therefore, and most importantly, if we are only disturbed by what we read, we lose the subtly and the larger context. I am writing to illuminate the larger picture, to outline the patterns of corruption, and then point the way to a solution. After all, this isn't about one unhealthy exchange between adult and child. This is about a pattern of secrecy, complacency, and disregard that has harmed far too many, for too long. It's about what happens to a social group when leaders fail us, and trust in society weakens.

If we are going to heal ourselves and our society, we have to stay focused on what matters in our process of recovery. We heal by naming the true nature of the disease and opening our minds to new thinking that can bring about a new way of doing things.

Useful Skills - Watching What People Do

This skill involves layers of seeing. Words are merely the nets and filters that allow us to catch a larger truth, so we can look at it more closely. Sometimes, though, words can block out the light and cast a shadow. So, we must learn to keep words in their right place; we can instead watch what people do.

Imagine you are a musician playing in the square dance band, on the slightly elevated stage above the dancers. Your hands know how to move along the strings (just as your eyes know how to glide over letters on a page). As one part of you plays the instrument or reads, another will be watching for patterns. You may notice one dancer in particular, but the skill here is to see the pattern of the whole as it moves. It's as simple as adjusting focus. Do the dancers form a clover? Is it a radial pattern or an actual square?

Choices made are the dance steps. We can pause at critical junctions in the upcoming Encounters and ask, *"What did they choose to do?"* Everything is a choice.

We also have to consider our own need for order, our *wanting to believe*. When it comes to schools, children, and the sectors of society where trust is crucial for health, we all want to believe our trust is warranted. It helps the world to make sense. It also is not easy to give up a previous stability in exchange for seeing clearly. But we are here to see more. So, we have to keep in check the part of ourselves that longs for reassurance. Just hold it suspended a while in moments of watching the dance.

As you track for *What People Do,* you can tell the *wanting to believe* part that you will meet back up once you have more information.

Hold on a moment here. I'm looking at something. I'll get right back to you, and we'll talk . . .

Tactics - D Words

It turns out, many of the tactics used to cover up the truth start with the letter D. So, while you're watching what people do, keep these maneuvers in mind.

Denial - the most basic, reflexive response: saying something is not true. Also, a psychological condition where someone will not admit to something painful (being in denial).

Diminishing - any effort to make the speaker of the truth feel or appear small: includes counter-attacks on character, minimizing the severity of an incident, putting one in a subordinate position in hopes of making the truth go away.

If you suddenly doubt your own perceptions or feelings, or question whether you have the right to address an issue at all, Diminishing may be at play.

Diversion - drawing attention away from the painful truth and toward an unrelated issue: often used to relieve the pressure of being seen or found out. This is also where blaming the speaker of a truth fits. Making it about the other person is a way to divert attention away from the real issue.

If you've ever brought a concern to someone, and suddenly found yourself talking about other things (possibly even *your* shortcomings), Diversion is likely at play.

Discrediting - an attempt to invalidate the truth by proving the speaker unworthy of belief or consideration: fault-finding that gets the one being held accountable 'off the hook' by confusing authority on the issue.

'You don't know what you're talking about', and *'Well, they're unstable, so you can't believe what they say'* are both Discrediting moves.

Defamation - by legal definition: any intentional false communication, either written or spoken, that decreases the respect, regard or confidence in which a person is held.

This is where it gets serious. The person afraid of the truth is willing to cause damage to another to protect their own comfort - even if that means lying to oneself or others.

For compassion, let's also remember the underlying D word:

Dissonance (from cognitive dissonance theory in psychology, investigated by Leon Festiger in 1957) a situation of conflicting attitudes, beliefs or behaviors that produces mental discomfort - leading to alteration in one of the attitudes, beliefs or behaviors, to reduce the discomfort and restore balance.

When there is inconsistency between attitudes and behaviors (dissonance), something must change to eliminate the dissonance. Saul McLeod from Simply Psychology says, "Notice that dissonance theory does not state that these modes of dissonance reduction will actually work, only that individuals who are in a state of cognitive dissonance will take steps to reduce the extent of their dissonance."

The first cause of Dissonance is identified as "Forced Compliance Behavior", when someone is forced to do something (publicly) that they (privately) really don't want to do. McLeod continues, "Forced compliance occurs when an individual performs an action that is inconsistent with his or her beliefs. The behavior can't be changed, since it was already in the past, so dissonance will need to be reduced by re-evaluating their attitude to what they have done."

Have you ever noticed someone altering their attitude about what they've done, in order to reduce their discomfort?

Apocalypse - The Unveiling

"The unseen is almost always
underlined with the unsaid."

— Viet Thanh Nguyen

November 2016 was the beginning of an Apocalypse. On November 9, I was sitting with my head in my hands, shoulders soft and pulsing as I wept at the enormity of totally unexpected news. It was generations of agony that coursed through me, and a concern for our species so vast that I could only surrender to the sadness.

My nine-year-old walked into the room to find me in this position, and said flatly, more as a statement than a question, "He won.".

Apocalypse is a Greek word meaning "the revelation" or "an unveiling or unfolding of things not previously known and which could not be known apart from the unveiling". For so many, though not for all, this conclusion revealed something shocking about our country. A bragging sexual assailant had made it to the highest office in the land. A man who unabashedly spread racist ideologies was becoming a decision-maker for a nation. If he hadn't secured the popular vote, the system had allowed him to reach this position of representing our country.

It all screamed a whole lot of questions. How many abuses of power had been quietly tolerated? How many justifications for misogyny or racial slurs? How many colleagues had bitten their tongue, and what inner conflicts kept them from speaking up? How prevalent was the idea that *boys will be boys*, and who did that serve?

So many people suddenly feared for their safety. People who were deemed "minority", yet accounted for a greater and greater majority of Americans, questioned whether work or school or recreation would now be safe. The autonomy and rights of women were now called into question on a much larger scale. This had been allowed to happen.

Personally, I had to ask: What is the connection between this event and my experience with Lawrence Academy?

To answer that, we first have to see the context leading up to the Apocalypse moment...

~ ~ ~

In the summer of 2016, I had travelled from Washington to Vermont with my child to fulfill a long-time dream of being in the Bread & Puppet Circus. There, we met up with a number of old friends, who easily decided without any suggestion, that we would get an AirBnB house and spend that weekend together in northern Vermont.

It was such bliss. Even after my exile and absence, these are the friends who have endured the changes of time and grown even more valuable each year. That weekend, we spent time in ways we might have happily dreamed up as teenagers. We had one big house, took turns making and cleaning up food, and watched after each other's children. I even extended the circle to include a friend I'd made on the west coast, who also happened to be from Massachusetts.

After dinner on our last night, we all started reminiscing, and I brought up the Pete Regis and Lawrence Academy thing. Some were casually milling around, the parents among us getting kids encouraged toward bed.

But, as soon as the topic arose, a solemn reverence set in, and everyone sat quietly back down. We all talked it over again. Yes, I'd given the speech, but what had really changed? They were proud of my accomplishment, but we sensed the larger issue was still unresolved. Friends being what they are, they knew I'd suffered for years without any rebalancing or compensation to my efforts, and this was wrong.

In this shared revisiting, we were all still rattled by the school leaders' choices. I know intuitively that many of these friends carried a pang of guilt, which wasn't theirs to bear, but still burdened their hearts. It was from knowing I'd been the one punished for speaking up and protecting others. We sat together amidst all of that awareness and emotion, as good old friends will.

I don't know how long it had been since I'd shared about that story in the physical presence of people who knew it so thoroughly. I didn't have to explain; they felt all of the subtleties with me. My body hadn't registered loving acceptance around it in maybe a decade or more. Most humbling was what my body then had to say about it...

We all had just one more day together before flights and drives home would begin. That morning, I noticed the skin under my left eye was periodically twitching and pulsing. I figured it was general nerves from the whole east/west tension in my life. I knew I'd been upset by touching in on that story while on the east coast again. I was patient about it during the transition day.

Yet, that physical sensation stayed with me all through the plane ride home and lingered for three full days afterward. I thought it would subside once I caught up on sleep and reoriented to life on the west coast. But, even three days after returning to Washington and all of my daily rhythms, the reminder persisted. I felt a certain kind of frustration. I was humbled, then impatient, and even annoyed. Perhaps I regarded it as a surprising frailty, despite all of my progress and triumphs. I believed I had come so far from all of that pain, that I had integrated so much. Wasn't I healed? I was nearly 40, after all.

But, my body remembered. Even when it doesn't fit our preconceived notions of timelines for recovery and bouncing back, we have to yield to that wisdom. Our body has the final word. I wonder now, as I look back at what transpired next... if my body actually knew that more - much more - was soon coming.

Checking In

Alright, dear readers, we are nearing the halfway point now. We are about to begin the high-speed wrangling, the fast-paced dance that brings light to what some desperately want to keep hidden. These motions play out between individuals and groups, yet are enactments of a larger truth. Watch for the larger truth. As you read, remember, the point of the wrangling is to reveal. Then, to create a new way forward.

Imagine we are running now through this tangle of brambles, like a maze that weaves a circuitous path all around an issue. At each turn, a new insight is shown to us. Some corners will reveal horrors that still the heart with a uniquely surprising pain and disappointment. There can be a heaviness of spirit as illusions come crashing down. The process of rebirth, of transformation, can be painful.

Yet, every tight and narrow place endured brings the promise of greater strength on the other side, as a new door inevitably opens. We will get there. The point is to pull ourselves through on a path of utmost clarity. Chances are, you may be reminded of similar constrictions. You may see yourself in the urges for control. You may wonder at times you've stayed silent and what opportunities were lost.

Keep heart. We meet now, in one moment of a story shared and exchanged. Decisions have been made, yet so many more await. You must decide for yourself about the tradeoffs you will make, the stands you will take - and when.

We're heading toward a solution to previous imbalances, and the future is brightest once we've braved the darkness.

I offer you my own definition to guide us through:

Corruption is the result of a series of 'going alongs' where one has been fooled or coerced into believing that all authority exists outside oneself. The antidote, therefore, is to know and trust ourselves. We can remember where true power lies and find the courage to question even the most benign of givens in any situation.

Ask & You Shall Receive
Part Two

Sybil sent an email in October that year, with a link to an article about Lawrence Academy:

Lawrence Academy asks sex misconduct victims to come forward

By **LOWELL SUN**
PUBLISHED: October 20, 2016 at 12:00 a.m. I UPDATED: July 11, 2019 at 12:00 a.m.

GROTON (AP) — Another Massachusetts boarding school says it's asking people to come forward if they have information about sexual misconduct.

Lawrence Academy in Groton is the latest in a string of schools to ask students and alumni for reports of current or past sexual abuse. Several elite boarding schools are dealing with such allegations, including Phillips Andover in Massachusetts, Pomfret in Connecticut and St. George's School in Rhode Island.

Dan Scheibe, Lawrence's head of school, sent a letter to the school community on Wednesday outlining how to report abuse.

In a statement on Thursday, he would not say whether the school had received any reports of abuse by school employees or students. He cited the privacy of those affected and the desire to preserve the integrity of the investigative process.

In May of 2016, The Boston Globe had released their Spotlight Investigation Report on abuse in New England Boarding Schools, titled, *"Private Schools, Painful Secrets"*[4]. The team reports:

"But now he [a former male student from the Fesseden School] is among a growing number of former students at New England private schools who are breaking their silence about sexual abuse by staffers. They are emboldened by a cascade of recent revelations about cases — many of them decades old — that were often ignored or covered up when first reported, and that school administrators still struggle to handle appropriately today."

Describing the scope of the problem - as it was known in 2016 - they continue:

"At least 67 private schools in New England have faced accusations since 1991 that staffers sexually abused or harassed more than 200 students, the Spotlight Team found through an examination of court cases, as well as interviews with alumni, relatives, school officials, and attorneys.

At least 90 lawsuits or other legal claims have been filed on behalf of the alleged victims, and at least 37 school employees were fired or forced to resign because of the allegations. In addition, nearly two dozen eventually pleaded guilty or were convicted on criminal charges of abusing children or related crimes.

The Globe also found 11 cases in which private school employees who were accused of sexual misconduct went on to work at other schools — an echo of the Catholic church scandal in which abusive priests were often moved to other parishes. At St. George's School alone, at least three staff members accused of misconduct have gone on to jobs where they faced subsequent

---

4 Globe Spotlight Team, May 6, 2016, https://www.bostonglobe.com/metro/2016/05/06/private-schools-painful-secrets/OaRI9PFpRnCTJxCzko5hkN/story.html

sexual misconduct allegations involving children… Large as those numbers of cases and victims are, they almost certainly underestimate the problem. No central database exists of allegations against private school employees, who are typically not required to be licensed. And schools often keep the reports confidential, even when payments are made to alleged victims."

By the time you read or hear this, the tally tops at least 300 students who endured abuse at over 100 schools. Globe reporters address the unique nature of private schools by saying:

"The schools, many with rich histories and famed alumni, have often struggled to balance the need to respond robustly to abuse allegations with a desire to guard their reputations. Historically, few allegations were reported to law enforcement, and many schools avoid publicizing them even today. Getting past the schools' reticence is a challenge; because these are private institutions, they are exempt from public records laws. And when the Globe sent surveys to 224 private schools on their experience with sexual misconduct allegations, only 23 — about 10 percent — chose to reply."

I read this in the wee hours of night in October 2016. I was so energized by that headline saying Lawrence Academy "Asks Sex Misconduct Victims to Come Forward", I could barely sleep that night. *'Funny,'* I thought, *'I've been coming forward since 1994…'*

I found this part in the article:

Share information about sexual misconduct at private schools with the Boston Globe Spotlight team by completing this request for information.

I did this, and by morning, I was ready for action. I called the Boston Globe and got a reporter on the phone to ask if they'd done any coverage of Lawrence Academy of Groton, MA. He said they had not. Then this nameless reporter told me, off the record, "You know, a lot of these schools are going to start putting out statements like this - to make it look like they're doing the right thing". Hearing that insight from an intelligent adult was huge for me. He, like I, saw the dual story very clearly.

The reporter then directed me to Mitchell Garabedian. He was the foremost lawyer working on these cases in the Boston area. Riding one wave of momentum to the next, I was soon on the phone with him. Our new, young puppy played at my feet as I spoke at the kitchen table. I was sleep-deprived and had dropped my child off at school less than an hour earlier. We'd brought this puppy home right after our Vermont trip, and we were all still learning one another. Suddenly, the puppy acted fearfully toward me, as if something other than me had overtaken my body. She seemed to recognize a threat and wanted to protect me from it. Yet, she couldn't find it; the threat was in me. I was reacting to something, and she was reacting to it. The clear alarm in her instinctive-animal system gave me new information about trauma and its reactivation.

Mitchell Garabedian asked me pointed questions and spoke quick details about charges and statutes of limitations. He said there was enough there for him to take the case. "It's evil, what they did to you.", Garabedian said. This gave me pause. Was he trying to play me into some game of, '*poor you!*' to win my trust? Whatever the cause, it inspired me to take a step back. "Evil" happens to be a word I do not tolerate, in speaking of others. I'll take all variety of profanity over "evil" or "hate". I am also not so easily hooked by us vs. them thinking.

He told me the whole process would take about 18 months. I would travel to Boston for a deposition, possibly also a hearing. He explained we would sue the perpetrator and leverage the risk to their reputation to account for their mishandling, even past the seven-year statute for suit against them. He told me we would settle "in the mid-six-figures", and he would take 1/3. Apparently, that is generous for the industry.

After this phone call, I had all the understanding of what it would mean to sue Lawrence Academy. I took a deep breath. Then, I called the school myself. *Ask, and you shall receive, Lawrence Academy*. I was thinking about the glossy publication of 2001 as I called and, "We'll be asking alumni for their input". Oh, yes. I had things to say. Now, '*Come forward*', you say?

Here I am.

You must be careful in what direction you begin to step on any important road. The placement of your feet at an auspicious juncture can define your ultimate outcome and destination. The phone rang, and soon a dry, middle-aged female voice spoke, *"Hello, Lawrence Academy."*. I told the secretary that I was calling in response to their statement and the article. In a very detached, apathetic voice, she asked for my name and phone number.

I felt a fierceness rising up from my chest. I heard myself growl in response, "No. I am calling to get information from *you*." I asked if there were any class action settlements underway. She said there were not. She tried again to take my name. I let that growl convey everything else I needed to communicate. "I said *I* am the one calling for information.". She grew flustered at someone inserting new steps into the same old dance. I got what clarity was available and hung up the phone.

~ ~ ~

Then, came the Apocalypse in November. The fervor of elections had peaked, and the waves of fear rolled across the country like so many amber waves of grain.

Intentions - The Amends Project

In my thirties, I became a mother, and very briefly, a wife. The man from the east coast and I had married during the pregnancy and divorced before our child turned three. I wasn't convinced yet, of the rightness of marriage for me, and he brought his own limitations. We'd made the more enduring commitment, though, and the strength of that promise remains.

Still, I loved a place, a region, and a town, and I lived my devotion to it. By November 2016, I was deep into my work in the world: making good on my promise to bring sexuality out from the shadows and into the healthy, joyful light where it belonged.

I was teaching what I called "Soulful Sexuality Education" to area private schools, focusing on middle school age and younger to send a new message early. I'd expanded my training at Planned Parenthood to include emotional intelligence and life navigation skills. Much of it was an echo of messages I'd given students in Groton, Massachusetts, at my speech in 2001.

I became the founder and Executive Director of a nonprofit called Rooted Emerging, offering puberty rite of passage programs. The message spoke to people, and I stayed busy supporting families, coordinating programs and events, and managing a growing group of adults who wanted to contribute to this vision. I naturally had started with a girls program, and on the urging of men and parents, I soon created a boys program.

Our Board had rich discussions on what this kind of offering meant, and the challenge of reaching young people for the experience. Women and daughters more easily signed up, while the young men resisted. It was the edge where a societal change needed to happen, yet patterns of embarrassment or avoidance were already so entrenched. While we didn't always fill slots for the full coming of age program, adults of all kinds started approaching me privately for support tending to these issues. I started consulting alongside teaching and leading the organization.

As a woman in my early 30s, I was always the youngest and least-formally-educated person in the Board room. Leadership came naturally, as fueled by my vision and the energy to bring that vision to life. To me, the heart of leadership is a willingness to do the right thing, speaking up, and living by integrity while doing so. More and more people came to be part of this vision, some by invitation and so many by attraction.

I did soon encounter the pretense of "status" on the west coast, reminiscent of the world of elites I'd grown among back east. Men with PhD's scoffed at needing to take direction from me, while doctors ruffled their feathers at not being the decision-maker in the group. Some sought to undermine me, even as many dozens encouraged all I worked to create. I suppose people everywhere can be susceptible to the desire to prove their worthiness by external signals.

~ ~ ~

Over the years of establishing myself as a professional in my hometown, I did have some funny, perspective-shaking moments. It was a kind of "coming to", where I'd suddenly look around and think, *'Wait, where was I?'* Like waking up from anesthesia, I would see that there was, indeed, this place I had left off. It was time now to pick back up... Mostly, I must admit, these moments came in witnessing the contrast to those around me.

Yes, my colleagues and I worked side-by-side, yet the course of their lives was entirely foreign to me. There was talk about grad school, the mortgage on their house in town, or their marriage of 10+ years. We related in so many ways through our shared work. Yet, I'd stand dumbfounded at the details of their lives. Then, I would see with sudden clarity, *'Oh, right, you didn't spend a decade running away from trauma.'*

I came to appreciate, as I stepped into my rightful place in my own life, that my reference on normal had existed on an entirely different plane of experience. My twenties were a blur of cross-country travels, surgeries, and learning to be independent in small towns along the west coast. That Bachelor's degree had finally come in the mail, just months before I gave birth at age 30.

I'd lived outside of a mainstream for over a decade, swimming this turbulent tributary upstream to some source for replenishing. I was one young woman reimagining the world at 70 mph, reconnecting with myself until I could find a way to live in this world, and in my body, well.

How many variant rivers there must be, for racial, immigrant, refugee, LGBTQ+, and more streams of human experience I can only imagine. Did they also feel themselves floundering against a current that might wash them to shore? I would have to climb so many hills of perspective to even glimpse those life paths. All of my peers now seemed to have moved smoothly along this steady current of growth and development, in a river that ran completely out of sight from my own.

I felt I breathed differently at this stage of life. Like I'd been kicked in the stomach at 16 in the headmaster's office, and then crawled through my life for about fifteen years. Finally, I stood up. Things looked different up here. But, at least I had gathered the strength to fully stand up.

We can set a course, and then find the boulder, in whatever form it takes. We have to redirect, and hopefully join up with cleaner, healthier waters as we go. Again, I count my time on the road as a blessing. But, oh, how life looked new from this shore. Perhaps, I now had seen the view from the rushing river, as well as the one from the bank besides. From the riverbank, I could finally build and give back in a whole new way.

~ ~ ~

During a follow-up conversation with Mitchell Garabedian's associate, he said to me in his east coast, tell-it-like-it-is, accent, "No offense, but you sound really together - and that's going to make it a tough sell, as a case."

More than once, Mitchell Garabedian had said to me, "I don't know if you know who I am..." He'd been the most successful lawyer in suing both the Catholic Church and New England Boarding Schools for these abuses for over thirty-five years. Both Ted Danson and Stanley Tucci had portrayed him in television and film about his career. Settlement amounts ranged from $2 million to individual plaintiffs, to $10 million from suit against a repeat offender priest, and upwards of $85 million in a case against the Archdiocese of Boston.

I had a decision to make. November had rolled by quickly, with world events on the political scale rushing all of us toward the necessity of adjustment and recovery. If we were going to move forward on this lawsuit, it was time to get going now.

Here's what I knew: I'd been on one, clear path of making things right for 25 years. I'd worked privately on that path, and no matter who joined me now, I would continue on that path undeterred.

What I didn't know: would a lawsuit get us further toward righting the bigger wrong?

What about the next kid who came forward with a report of abuse? (I was astute and seasoned enough to know, there would be another kid) I saw the intricate web of secrecy and silencing around every one of these incidents. Would suing the school alter the course of business-as-usual? It was the web that needed dismantling.

With a high-profile lawyer behind me, could I get better results? I thought of Steve Hahn telling me in 2006 that he was headmaster again, but in a new state. I weighed the value of keeping my story private as I had. Then, I thought of Steve Hahn telling me back in the '90s that they had acted "within the law". Something bigger had to step in on this. I felt a draw to finally having an ally on my side, where I'd always been so alone and screaming into the abyss before.

Voices of all kinds were resounding with me now. Women were calling bullshit on the way men had handled and mistreated them - and those who loved them cried in rage at the decades of stored pain. All the effects of too much complacent silence were staring at us from within an oval office. The ills of corruption and patriarchy were a big problem before us, asking for a very big response.

I was ready to go big, yet there were so many unknowns. So, I set an intention. I would resume my efforts now if we could truly make amends. This move had to repair and mend the fractures that were so vast around all of us now.

This would be The Amends Project.

On the morning of my 39th birthday, I called Mitchell Garabedian's office in Boston. I said I was ready to retain him to represent me in a lawsuit against Lawrence Academy of Groton, Massachusetts.

Crossroads & Divergences

January 2017 brought the largest, global scale protests in human history. Women's Marches were held in 81 countries around the globe, with an estimated seven million demonstrators. Six hundred seventy-three protests on all seven continents on the planet. People from every corner of our world showed up on their streets in support of women's rights and bodily sovereignty.

By August 2017, it was time for the attorney's office to send a demand letter to Lawrence Academy. "This gets their attention, and starts the process.", Mitchell Garabedian told me.

His office did everything by paper mail, which made for a slower, if more confidential, process. So, one day in August, I found at my PO Box the draft of our Demand Letter.

I was jarred as I read it. Right in the first official paragraph, it listed all these psychoses I'd never spoken of, many of which I just didn't identify with. Some of the impacts of my suffering were there, yes. But, this was not me by a long shot. I also knew I was not going to be dishonest in the hopes of getting more money.

I called to discuss the letter, first getting the associate, and then Garabedian, on the phone. He soon realized I was fully noncompliant with the letter as it stood. Mitchell rapidly, and then furiously fielded my objections. His first response was smug, "Well, we'll have you come to Boston for a 3-hour psychiatric evaluation, and that will help". Apparently, they had people they could count on to dig up some verifiable 'crazy' on clients. The implication was - I was not the authority on my inner world - but someone else could be.

My approval was needed to send this letter (let's remember he was, after all, working for me). The process was not going as he had wanted. Most of all, I noticed the issue of exploitation was front and center. Let's review.

The groundskeeper at Lawrence Academy had tried to exploit my body for a diseased, personal gain. Then, the school had exploited my education and safety in the world to protect their reputation. Now, I was being asked to let these people exploit my psyche in hopes of even larger financial settlement.

Garabedian fell into his 'interrogation/cross-examination' mode, seeming to forget that I was his client and not an opposing party in the courtroom. "Have you ever felt that way? Did you ever think that way in the past?" I answered honestly, and he grew increasingly impatient and combative.

I remembered my intention about The Amends Project and knew I had to gauge my next steps accordingly. In the short-term, playing the game to get some prize can be efficient, if unethical. But, this was a long-game. I knew that. I wasn't going to lose sight of right and wrong in this moment, or make myself part of something that was indifferent to the distinctions.

It matters how we get there.

I questioned why there was a hefty paragraph on my "damages" and barely a clear sentence on their unethical choices. He brushed that aside as legal strategy. "When do they admit to the cover-up?" I asked. He said that wasn't
part of it. Then, he continued to escalate and push harder. At the peak of his frustration, Garabedian said sharply, "You know, this thing you went through... it really gave you some *control* issues".

"Well, that's insulting.", I said in slow-motion, 'Oh, no you don't' tone into the phone. "And as for what I went through," I fumed, "I tell *you* how this impacted me - **not** the other way around."

Garabedian excused himself and let the associate take it from there. He and I calmly worked to edit and revise a list that was true enough for me and punchy enough for their purposes. The law office set the demand at 2 million dollars, put that letter in the mail to Lawrence Academy, and the process had begun.

~ ~ ~

I quietly came to a place of inner resolve that my dignity was what mattered most in this process. I mailed a letter asking Mitchell Garabedian for an apology. Many weeks went by before I could get him on the phone. When we did speak, I asked for the apology. He would not give one. I told him I couldn't proceed, then - and he agreed we shouldn't work together.

That was that.

There can be many lonely moments on the road to staying true to oneself. It is a very unique kind of loneliness, though. You might miss the beauty initially, but that particular sadness always drifts away on the next strong breeze. What's left, beneath the winds sweeping the old away, is an enhanced resolve and strength like bedrock that is unshakable.

I stepped off that path and faced a whole new kind of unknown.

Integration - East & West

"Man cannot discover new oceans
unless he has the courage
to lose sight of the shore."

— Lord Chesterfield

I spent some time mourning the loss of what I believed would be powerful backup. Slowly, I came to understand, there is no switching positions and gaining progress in a game of win-and-lose with patriarchy. Having a big lawyer to fight a big corruption was not the advantage I was seeking. No matter where you stand in that paradigm, it's still the same game.

I would have to initiate a new game altogether.

Patriarchy is a social construct of male dominance and an ideology of authority and social privilege as relegated to males.

Phillipe Leonard Fradet, writer at The Body is Not an Apology, describes Patriarchy in 2018 this way:

1. a lack of reflectiveness; not putting effort into questioning social norms, or how one's actions affect others.

2. competition; the tendency for men to be in competition with each other and needing to see themselves as better than others in nearly every aspect of their lives.
3. Patriarchy seeks to protect a status quo; an exaggerated dislike of discomfort, especially as it threatens to take one out of their comfort zone; and
4. an urge to stay comfortable at all costs
5. These and other attributes he sums up to a toxicity

He concludes that these modern qualities of patriarchy make things worse for those subjected to the subordination or oppression - and for the men who seem to benefit from it.

Fradet says, "Men are hurt by their own dedication to toxic, patriarchal masculinity by allowing themselves to hurt others.".

I knew the world of men. I had grown there more completely than in a world of women. I care about this as a lover of men and someone who wants better for all of us.

Though we fundamentally disagree on approach, I give respect to Mitchell Garabedian for the immense ground he covered in reconciling institutional child abuse. Before his decades of effort, the norm had been to quietly settle with parishioners out of court, with settlements capping out at $25,000 because of the limit referred to as "charitable immunity". This means nonprofit charities - like churches and some private schools - are immune from legal fines exceeding $25,000. Of course, those limits were likely set from the healthy place of *never imagining* that employees and priests would be abusing children within their own membership.

In the 2015 Spotlight movie (where actor Stanley Tucci plays Mitchell Garabedian), reporter Sacha Pfieffer hears of the settlements being offered by Garabedian's predecessor, Eric McLeash, at around $25,000. She says, aghast, "Twenty-five thousand dollars?! That's the fine for child abuse?"

Mitchell Garabedian has brought this painful legacy to a much higher level of reckoning and justice. He produced the kinds of settlements that actually account for the damages caused by these large institutions. His career and devotion brought profound healing for many. I tip my hat to all he achieved in his time.

I am simply saying it is a new time - time to address these situations in a whole new way.

~ ~ ~

The weeks passed in a quiet daze for me, while news of Harvey Weinstein and more and more Hollywood actresses' accusations painted a picture. Like Weinstein, Lawrence Academy groundskeeper, Peter Regis was formulaic; he had a pattern of behavior he repeated with young women to see how far he could get. He was a predator in the same way Weinstein had been. Now, that pattern was showing itself to the world through the high-profile entertainment industry.

On a personal level, I enjoyed a professional success that fall when I was awarded the "Kickass Single Mom" grant for my work in sexuality education and youth rites of passage. I'd recently completed a 10-month Professional Coach Certification training, and encompassed all of my works into a social enterprise called Love & Truth Rising. The announcement read, "I chose this month's winner because her mission is so very apropos to this chapter of women's empowerment" and referenced Weinstein and the web of silent complacency around this man. The honor included a $1,000 award and an hour-long interview on the "Like a Mother" podcast.

We didn't even talk about my long journey with Lawrence Academy during the interview. She drew the connection between my current life's work and what was happening with Harvey Weinstein, and the #MeToo movement, as I was encouraging young people to own their sexual natures. When she asked how I got into this work, I said simply, "There are many threads to the story.". I stayed focused on my Gramma and my lifelong role of guiding and protecting youth.

For my first national audience interview, I was intensely anxious about exposure on such a large scale. I am a private person, willing to put myself out there for a cause. I had done this in my small city of Bellingham, Washington, many times. Yet, there is another unique thread in my life's experience: I had never been on social media. The whole phenomenon passed me by like some wave I missed while traveling the roads of this country.

Often, I would reemerge into society to feel suddenly jarred by technological developments around me. I walked onto the campus of the University of Oregon one day in my mid-twenties and saw young people talking on cell phones as they walked! No eye contact with passers-by. A whole new body language in the world. I was stunned and thought, *'Who are they talking to?!'*

It was the same with social media. I remember the season in 2007, when my good, long-time friends started emailing to ask me to join this thing called Facebook. I looked at the site and felt absolutely no draw, and even a bit eerie about it. I found it unsettling that you would let your private conversations become public viewing material. Likely, my history of enduring stalking by Peter Regis contributed to the discord. I saw that people were 'counting' how many friends they had for a public tally, too. "No, thanks," I would respond to each request. "But, rest assured, I am your friend in the real world."

This was the main reason I didn't identify with the #MeToo movement, much as I have been reassured, and hold great respect for everything it signifies in our world. Breaking silences that protect a wrongdoer for the sake of repair is always worth celebrating. The platform where it all unfolded was just too foreign to me. The second reason is that my impactful experience wasn't really sexual abuse - it was institutional abuse.

So, I braved a New York City-based podcast interview that fall, just before the holidays. All the while, I still had no idea what would come next in my Amends Project effort.

~ ~ ~

As a youth advocate and Executive Director of Rooted Emerging, I was a member of the Whatcom Prevention Coalition in Bellingham, Washington, and attended regular meetings. This group consisted of educators, counselors, school administrators, nonprofit leaders of all kinds, and various health professionals - all focused on healthy youth development. Each meeting focused on a different theme, with members contributing their knowledge on subjects in turn and leading discussions. After many weeks of staring blankly into the unknown, something of an answer showed up during a Prevention Coalition meeting.

A woman named Shasta Cano-Martin came in to give a presentation on Peacemaking Circles. She invited Coalition members to their monthly healing circle on the Lummi Nation, the tribal lands just north of town. Shasta was Executive Director of the Lummi C.E.D.A.R Project, a Native American nonprofit focused on youth development and leadership on the Lummi Reservation. I'd heard many times of her work, as people recognized a kinship with my coming of age programs at Rooted Emerging. The project focused on Community health, Elders, Education, Drug-free, Alcohol-free, Respect (CEDAR).

It was here I learned of Saroeum Phoung and Restorative Justice. As she spoke about bringing people together to honestly face the harms caused in a spirit of acknowledgment and respect, everything I needed to accomplish in my private Amends Project suddenly made sense. Cano-Martin spoke of Saroeum as her mentor and mentioned his consulting business, Point One North. I excitedly took notes for research later. She said he had worked with gangs in Boston for alternate resolution and in King County (Seattle, Washington) Juvenile Court to bring circle practice into jails and schools.

I was completely elated. Not only did this man's approach ring true for the goals of actually creating Amends, but he had connections on both sides of the country - Boston and Seattle. My two geographical points of contact and action! My east and my west were suddenly coming together, and I knew he was my next, true ally on this path.

I reached out by phone, and Saroeum received me warmly, through his association with Shasta. I told him where I was in my process with Lawrence Academy, and he was clear and capable in crafting next steps with me. I was awash with gratitude. Saroeum gave freely of his time, squeezing me into existing appointments and never asking for compensation for his efforts. I began preparing to engage with Lawrence Academy leaders in a whole new way.

~ ~ ~

I did some research and found images and videos of current headmaster, Dan Scheibe. I recognized that he was younger - maybe within a decade of my age. He seemed humble and personable compared to Steve Hahn. Following Hahn's departure in 2002 (after my December 2001 speech), I learned that Lawrence Academy had hired a man named Scott Wiggins. He had resigned a year before his contract expired in 2012 because of a controversy surrounding the football team and misuse of financial aid.

Sanctions were handed down from the Independent School League for violations, the details of which were also kept secret, yet involved financial aid. Boston.com reported confusion around the violations in 2011, which angered some.

"Lawrence Academy, through director of communications David Casanave, would only say, "Under advice of counsel, we're not going to comment on underlying issues that led to the sanctions."

Paul Lannon was attorney for Lawrence Academy at the time, and this "say nothing" approach was familiar to me when I found this.

"The school's no comment aggravated one graduate who was e-mailed the statement.

"'To not fully disclose what is going on is just the wrong way to treat your alumni and the rest of the school community,' wrote the graduate, who wished to be anonymous, in an e-mail.

"ISL coaches and athletic directors were told not to comment on the sanctions."

Silence does not protect people who have suffered, nor does it protect those who have done wrong. To impose silence on others is its own form of abuse.

The most recent article on Wiggins and the football scandal concluded, "the league demanded accountability regarding how it handles financial aid, particularly to student-athletes.". So, a decade after my speech to expose the school in 2001, another Lawrence Academy headmaster was implicated in abusing financial aid. It seemed, one leader quietly ducking away did not solve a persistent problem. Scott Wiggins' resigned the same way Steve Hahn did in 2011. Then, in 2012, Dan Scheibe took the post.

~ ~ ~

"What is society? ... It's a contract we sign as human beings amongst each other. We sign a contract with each other as people, whether it's spoken or unspoken, where we say, 'amongst this group of us we agree on common rules, common ideals, and common practices that are going to define us as a group' . . . And as with most contracts, the contract is only as strong as the people who are abiding by it. . . There is no contract if law and people in power don't uphold their end of it. . . We need people at the top to be the most accountable, because they are the ones who are basically setting the tone and the tenor for everything that we do in society. It's the same way we tell parents to set an example for their kids. . . the same way you tell teachers to set an example for their students. . . If you lead by example there is a good chance that people will follow that example you have set."

— Trevor Noah

I sent a paper letter to Lawrence Academy in Groton, Massachusetts in late 2017, asking the school to settle with me out of court. I proposed they give 45% of Mitchell Garabedian's demand, or to settle with me at 35% and include a Restorative Justice process. I received a curt letter back from attorney Paul Lannon, with Dan Scheibe's name attached, vaguely disregarding my claims and asking, "Do you have a lawyer?".

I responded by letter to Daniel Scheibe on January 9, 2018, "Because of my interest in utilizing a Restorative Justice approach, I am in the process of shifting legal representation." I later received an additional letter from Dan Scheibe, where he actually wrote, "I am sure that you are above the monetary approach to settlement". I replied again by written letter:

February 1, 2018

Daniel Scheibe
Lawrence Academy

Greetings Dan,

Thank you for your quick reply. I am glad to hear that you are selecting a Restorative Justice path, and have willingness to address monetary compensation. I agree this is the best approach.

Seeing as you did not specifically select one of the two options posed, let me reiterate here what I need, moving forward:

1. the ability to select my own representation, within the Restorative Justice format
2. commitment of all parties involved to adhere to the date of February 28, 2018 for session
3. a minimum of $700,000 compensation (with legal fees) or $600,000 (without legal fees)

Money is not beneath the goals of this process; it is an essential component. Consider that I live the realities of my derailed college path and postponed adult career every single day. I live it on a financial level, as much as I have lived it on emotional and physical levels.

To be sincere, reparations must be made on a financial level. I understand that statutes of limitation exist to protect would-be defendants. Yet, we all have to acknowledge, over-protection of the school's interests was at the root of this atrocity to begin with.

When it comes to protection of interests today, the party whose needs take precedence here is mine.

. . . I am including a brief overview of losses and injuries suffered as a result of the school's handling: the neglect, exile, intimidation and psychological abuse. This is not a comprehensive Impact Statement, but a prelude, which justifies the figures I present to you...

Keep in mind, the process of true repair - while it may be healthy and restorative - is not meant to be clean and easy. I ask that you prepare yourself to put some serious 'skin in the game' and ready your willingness to do the real work.

Walking this path with you, outside of what I believe to be a destructive, unethical approach, requires a measure of trust. I am asking you to prove worthiness of that trust by meeting these initial criteria. If I see that these are taken seriously, with written confirmation by mail by February 15, 2018, I will be happy to proceed with you in this way.

I look forward to your response.

Sincerely,

Vanessa Osage

~ ~ ~

I had sat down one afternoon and begun calculating all of my expenses and losses from the incidents at Lawrence Academy. It took many days to complete an accurate accounting in my spare time. I factored in counseling, surgeries, travel to and from Groton, Massachusetts, in 2001. I called hospitals and asked for rates on procedures at the time I had them. I produced medical records through numerous phone calls. I also accounted for lost wages and earnings over time. I was doing my own research to represent myself. The number I came to was $640,500. Knowing this, I had more confidence suggesting an amount for compensation - even if it was far less than Mitchell Garabedian's $2 million demand.

~ ~ ~

I continued to stay in touch with Saroeum Phoung as I kept letters moving east to west, back and forth to Lawrence Academy by mail. Soon, it was time for Saroeum to speak with Dan Scheibe and attorney Paul Lannon himself, to prepare us all for a Circle process. Dan Scheibe had sent a letter confirming the date of February 28, 2018. This timing was crucial for me, as it was extraordinarily difficult to leave my day-to-day life for that kind of trip; it was the only window I had. Dan Scheibe and Paul Lannon agreed to this date.

I decided to talk to Dan myself first. If we were going to meet in circle, we needed to start coordinating details more quickly. Late February was fast approaching. With written agreement on all sides, Dan and I set a date for a first phone call. He told me his assistant, Libby Margraf, would be joining in.

One point stands out so clearly from that first live conversation. Dan Scheibe was careful and restrained as he spoke. Libby was mostly silent. I was focused and alternately clear and rattled. At one point, I said, "I need a minute. This is hard for me because it has been so traumatizing". Dan Scheibe softened his tone and said, "I can assure you, you are safe here. You are safe with Libby and me". He gave assurances for my safety.

In so many ways, Dan wanted me to know that things were better now. Lawrence Academy was a new kind of place, and he was a new kind of headmaster. Everything had changed, he said. Beneath all of our communications was a message from Dan Scheibe that I had nothing to worry about; everything was different and better now.

I wanted to believe. I truly did, want to believe.

Quick, She's Coming!

Plane tickets were purchased. Agreements were created and sent to all parties. Sareoum had phone calls with Dan Scheibe, Paul Lannon, and myself. A timeline was laid out and agreed upon. Effective Circle processes require a minimum of three days, Saroeum explained. So, we had confirmed February 28, March 1 and March 2, 2018. Steve Hahn would be there. Dan Scheibe, Paul Lannon, Libby Margraf, and I, along with Saroeum, would participate. Everything was set.

Then, we faced a sudden scheduling conflict. Saroeum had something come up which could not be moved. He asked, could we postpone even just a few weeks? Sadly, I could not. Dan Scheibe and Paul Lannon were eager to delay, as they wanted more time to prepare. This set my instincts off into heightened alertness. I knew what that meant. I was going way out on a limb to even walk through this new kind of road with the school. They had every advantage to manipulate the situation to their benefit. This was like Steve Hahn telling me in 1997, 1998, 1999, 2000... "Pete's going to retire soon.", or "Sure, I will see what I can do.", all while *nothing* changed.

I could not afford to take the risk of losing the cohesion we'd created to that point. I was about to fly east to try to resolve this long-standing issue out of court. I had to carry on. I was so grateful to Saroeum for his willingness to prepare us and to line up his travel to Boston with mine. He suggested we would fly from Seattle together and catch up on the plane. But the timing fell out of sync, right at the last moment, and threatened to unravel the process.

I told Dan Scheibe and Paul Lannon that I would travel alone to Boston, and we would walk through the process that Saroeum had so carefully laid out. Both men acknowledged my message. The travel date arrived, and then I was on my way . . .

~ ~ ~

A friend had dropped me off at the small Bellingham airport at 3 am, the morning of February 27, 2018. I would fly to Seattle and catch a connector flight to Boston. I was the full 90 minutes early to my flight, and it was a ghost town in there. I was one of maybe three travelers who sleepily roamed the halls of the airport. I checked my one bag, lay down on a bench with my carry-on, and rested while an employee vacuumed nearby. Over the subtle hum of the vacuum, I did not hear my boarding call. I actually missed the flight out of Bellingham, Washington. My bag went on to Boston, but I was stuck at home, figuring out how the hell to catch up.

Now, I generally like to travel, but what ensued next was a day of pure hell. I started calling for arrangements to catch a different flight from Seattle to Boston. I considered taking a bus or finding a ride to Seattle, but both proved futile. I would miss the connector flight either way. When I did get to Seattle, I had to be searched at the airport check point. The airport personnel were so cold and mechanical; it frightened me. What was happening with people in this country? My anxiety over what I was about to do, entirely on my own, reached a peak, and I broke down crying at Sea-Tac.

When I finally got to Boston, it was after 10 pm, making for a 16 hour day at that point. Everything was closed and quiet at Logan Airport. I could see my bag stored inside a glass-walled room, but everything was locked. I tried to arrange for an employee to open to door via those blue courtesy phone, but no response anywhere. I'd met the other ghost town on the east coast now, after odd stretches of hurry up and wait all day long. It seemed like ghosts of the corrupt and inhumane rolled around my feet like tumbleweeds on either side of this valiant effort to take a higher road. Worlds collided all around me.

I drove the old, childhood-familiar highways in Massachusetts in the dark to a new plaza on Route 119 in Littleton - one that hadn't existed in 2001 - and found the hotel. When I rang the bell near 1 am on February 28, a bleary-eyed attendant appeared and gave me a plastic key card. Then, he handed me a sealed envelope with Lawrence Academy insignia in the corner. In my exhaustion, I figured it was paperwork to sign. I stumbled up to my room and into sleep.

~ ~ ~

Sleep truly makes everything better, and I woke with some calm, but a live-wire energy for what lay ahead. I slowly washed my travel clothes in the sink and wrung them out to dry in the shower. I had about two hours until the start of our process. I would have to go in my soft pants and T-shirt. But, I was rested and deliberate. Then, I unfolded the mystery of the envelope . . .

It was a full-page, typed letter, signed by Dan Scheibe. I scanned over the flowery language I came to expect in all formal statements, trying to find the meat of what he was saying. Then, I found it. He said that **he had cancelled the Restorative Justice process** - but that he and Libby would be happy to meet with me in his office.

I was enraged! I had flown all the way across the country on his word and agreement. We had done all this work to get to this moment. Did he really think I would just say, "ok, never mind"?! I got Dan on the phone and railed, "I don't know what you are thinking, but you need to get EVERY one of those players back into this process Right Now and confirm with me within the hour. Is that clear?!" I recognized my own, not-fucking-around mama voice bellowing at this man I was still yet to meet.

He paused, and soon eked out a, "Yes, it's clear.". I continued, "Things were supposed to be better now, and this is No Different than how things have been handled all along. I trusted you to be good to your word, and you need to honor that word NOW." Scheibe then said something about Paul Lannon wanting facilitators. "Then, I'll find facilitators. You get everyone back on track, and I will arrange facilitators of my choosing.". I continued, "How could you not talk to me about this before I flew to Boston?!"

He said, "You were traveling.". I countered, "Yes, I was traveling - and I was on the phone numerous times throughout the day. You could have contacted me. That is NO excuse.".

We quietly hung up, and I got to work.

I did a search for "Restorative Justice facilitators Boston" and found something I somehow hadn't seen before. There was a Center for Restorative Justice at Suffolk University in Boston. I read the bio of a woman who had studied sociology and focused on gender equality issues. I wanted her right away. I called and explained that I'd traveled from Seattle for a Circle process that day, and I needed facilitators as soon as possible. I said I was prepared to do this on my own, so students or interns were fine. I just needed someone.

The student who answered the phone took down all of my information and promised that I would hear from Carolyn Boyes-Watson, the Director of the Center, as soon as possible.

I got a call from Dan with updates, saying he could have everyone gathered again by tomorrow. "We are missing a whole day.", I said, exaggerating the impacts of his decision. He suggested I come over to Lawrence Academy to meet and sign the Confidentiality Agreement that afternoon. I'd made a number of various calls, left messages, and reached a waiting point. So, I agreed.

~ ~ ~

It's amazing how places can look increasingly smaller and less impressive as you continually revisit them. I walked into that school building, all white and colonial, and felt only utter annoyance at the realities surrounding my walking up those steps. I had suggested we hold the Circle in the headmaster's office (which was now the Admissions office) so I could enjoy a "do-over" on their response to me. I believed having a new experience in the place where I had, 1. played headmaster, 2. been tricked into a meeting with Department of Social Services and, 3. received the debilitating news that I would not be coming back would offer the greatest possible healing.

After two hundred years, though, what is it to truly change the nature of a man-made place?

~ ~ ~

Dan Scheibe looked utterly terrified when he first held my gaze inside the school-house. My own animal nature recognized that true power did not exist here, only illusions and a fearful attempt at deflecting any too-clear gaze. Libby Margraf was pleasant and distanced in a way that suggested she was only there to bear witness. I was wearing my line-dried soft cotton T-shirt and black yoga pants as my only option. My own lack of appropriate dress only seemed to accentuate the 'Fuck it' nature of the moment. I am here, bearing witness to both of you, and to all of this. There is a nakedness in my approach, as much as a disregard for any pretense. I see every bit of this from an unguarded place, and I see you without your attempted guard, as well.

We began to speak, and I said, "This is awkward since I have no real business with the two of you.". As we got into the details of the issue at hand, and how we would address it, Dan grew nervous and jumpy. He was eager to have the confidentiality agreements signed right away (the same agreement he would later violate, by sharing sensitive sexual abuse details in a public statement without consent). Before this, though, numbers were briefly discussed, and he quickly implied that my - and therefore, Mitchell Garabedian's - numbers reflected much more severe levels of abuse.

I said, "Well, we have to account for the impact of the school's decision to keep him employed and revoke my financial aid.". Dan Scheibe then said what would become important, prophetic words, **"We're not exactly in agreement about that."**. It was as if I'd finally met that ghost of corruption, which had been foreshadowed all through my surreal travels the day before. To this, I replied forcefully, "How could there be disagreement? That's the easiest thing to prove. Look at any yearbook from 1994-95, and you'll see he was still there, and I was gone."

~ ~ ~

To calm my system and get perspective, I left the Lawrence Academy campus and drove to the nearby Nagog Hill, my very favorite place on the east coast. There, the land soothed me. I walked in silence to the pond and back, tracing the steps I had taken so many times in 2006, the year I lived on the east coast after my most major surgery. From that place, I could remember the broader goals of what I was working to achieve, even amidst the fallout from their latest tactic.

Then, in that calm, comforting place, my phone rang and showed an unknown 617 number. I answered, and it was Carolyn Boyes-Watson. "I understand you flew in from the west coast and need facilitators tomorrow, is that correct?". Yes, I told her. I then went on to give her the long-version of the story: from confronting the child molester in 1994, to losing my financial aid, being sent away, the speech, the attorney, the agreement for the Restorative Justice Circle, and finally, this moment.

She spoke deliberately, with a reverence, and said, "Well, first, I want to celebrate your conviction in persisting on this effort for so long". She continued, "Normally, I require much more preparation time, but if the alternative is you doing this on your own, we will think of something.". I was relieved and grateful to connect with her. I noticed my encounters seemed to alternate between the dodgy, fearful, and deceptive to the clear, honorable, and high-minded. Like driving across the country, east to west - my whole system breathed a sigh of relief.

Paradigms Collide

"Vulnerability transforms you.
You can't be in the presence of a truly vulnerable,
honestly vulnerable person and not be affected.
I think that's the way we are meant to be
in the presence of one another."

— Father Richard Rohr

Miraculously, by 7 am the next morning, March 1, 2018, two young women from the Center for Restorative Justice at Suffolk University were walking into the hotel lobby in Littleton, Massachusetts, to meet me and prepare for the process ahead. Both admitted they had never even sat in on a process of this scale. Yet, they were focused and rising to the moment with every bit of strength and determination. We had the framework created by Saroeum and my readiness to lead the process if need be.

I also signed a Confidentiality Agreement for the Restorative Justice Circle that day, the one created by Saroeum Phoung. There are places where I strongly believe in the value of confidentiality; it is a core tenet of my work with youth, adults, and families. When people share intensely personal things with me, I hold those details in a vault. I also understand the places where confidentiality is not appropriate. I know when it exists as a secrecy shield to hide the facts of wrongdoing by others.

So, to honor my word, I can share little about what unfolded in the old headmaster's office. I will honor my word on principle, though, even when others don't.

Here is what I can say: what was originally agreed upon as a three-day process - two full days, plus one half-day - was abbreviated to just one day with a long break. Steve Hahn was present for the first part of the day, along with Dan Scheibe, Paul Lannon, Libby Margraf, the two facilitators, and myself. After lunch, we agreed to discuss the repairs and response. For this portion of the day, Steve Hahn chose to not be present.

I sat with all of these people, feeling eternally that I was fighting a beast alone. Still, the honesty of the situation emerged before us. I cried, and I shook at times when I spoke. I clenched my belly unconsciously in pain as I recounted vivid moments along the way. We all set parameters at the beginning. I said I might swear, but would not swear at anyone directly, nor would I call names. At one point, many hours in, I screamed my objections to Steve Hahn. Struggling to channel that rage into something measured and coherent, I ratcheted the energy down enough to say, "I hope screaming is o.k.". Meanwhile, students shuffled their feet outside the doors of the old headmaster's office.

No agreements were reached on liability by the school or amounts for compensation. Liability can be determined in a Restorative Justice process; these men chose not to claim it. To honor myself, I said I could not leave that room until we had some written agreement for an offer of settlement. It was like wandering into the dragon's lair, naked and alone, while scores of vultures watched in wait. Dan and Paul scratched a handwritten promise to provide an offer within the week. Even with that in hand, I could not leave the room before any others. Call it primal. I had a profound need to see as much as possible, to make sense of it as best I could while I was there.

I watched every single player leave the room - and I sat with the silence that lingered once they left.

I watched the way Paul Lannon looked at and regarded Dan Scheibe as he walked out the door. Recall from the Boston.com article, "Under advice of counsel, we're not going to comment on underlying issues that led to the sanctions.". Paul Lannon was creating a legacy for himself by pressuring people into silence. Paul self-consciously addressed Dan, the way an actor might - after the costumes were put away backstage, and an audience member awkwardly lingered for the after-show departure. They were both in and out of character. In my perception, there was no camaraderie, no respect in that gaze. I felt entirely unnerved by what I saw between them as he walked out the door. "Bye, Dan.", he said from a distance at the threshold, almost for show. "See ya, Paul.", Dan Scheibe called back.

I was 40 years old when I sat alone in that room, breathing in the silence after a full day of so much spoken, and these people gathered for such a short time. My mind processed the faces I'd observed, sometimes sincere and present - other times seeming calculated and controlled. My body calmed down after many storms had passed. All the while, I was calmly noticing the chipped white paint, the cracked and faded moldings around old windows. It all looked like some relic of a dying vestige to patriarchy. I watched all those sensations - internal moments in my mind's eye, and external details of a strange, fabricated environment - all fading away from me, like miles along the interstate.

~ ~ ~

"Responsibility is the thing people dread most of all.
Yet it is the one thing in the world that develops us,
gives us manhood or womanhood fiber."

— Frank Crane

March 9, 2018

Dear Vanessa,

…we disagree as to Lawrence Academy's financial responsibility to your current situation. As promised, we discussed your experiences and request for monetary compensation with the Executive Committee of the Board of Trustees. We presented your case thoroughly and with care as you represented it in writing and in person.

[why do men keep trying to "represent" me, when I am obviously representing myself?]

In our view, and in the Board's view, the money you are seeking is not commensurate with the wrongful conduct at issue or with a reasonable extension of the school's responsibility.

The board has authorized me to offer you $25,000 in full and final settlement. This offer is contingent upon the signing of a formal written agreement that includes a general release of legal claims, confidentiality as to the amount and terms of the agreement, and no admission of legal liability… Please let us know if you accept the offer and we will send you a draft agreement that you may review.

Sincerely,

Dan Scheibe
Head of School

Mar 9, 2018, 11:00 AM

Dan,

This settlement amount is simply not sufficient. It doesn't even scratch the surface of reimbursing for basic health expenses I have endured. I was already clear that even that minimal amount would be insulting. This reflects to me what an institution is willing to release, with absolutely minimal impact on itself.

It is not sufficient and I cannot accept.

I suppose this is the folly of asking the descendants of a crime what they think their group currently needs to do. That decision truly should not lie in the hands of the school alone.

This reminds me of asking a child what they think they should do to make up for breaking a neighbor's windows with a ball. The child says, "fifty cents?". There needs to be another authority looking on this besides the one that carries responsibility...

I will return to this later today, when I have time.

Thank You,

Vanessa

Sybil, as always, had been my primary source of contact and support throughout my trip east. I knew it would be a fast and furious visit, with only this business to attend. So, she was the one person outside Lawrence Academy officials I made time to see. We stayed in touch by phone leading up to the Circle process, and we met for dinner once it was all done.

She listened to me exhale all the various highs and lows of the wild experience so far, as we enjoyed Thai food in that new, surreal plaza in Littleton. We relaxed into a late evening as we'd done so many times, for over twenty five years. Her characteristic humble, head lowered in contemplation posture in the motel room brought me all the familiar comfort of an old friend. We talked until it was late, obviously past the point of coherence, and said goodnight. I flew out of Boston in the morning.

Sybil called during my extended layover in San Francisco, en route home to Washington. I'd arranged it intentionally, to reset my system before diving back into my busy life at home. I knew I would be uniquely rattled, and I finally had the wisdom to account for this re-regulation time. I'd slept twelve hours the night before in my AirBnB in the east bay. So, I was already lucid by the time she called.

She told me that she'd visited her mom, Michelle Johnson, after our dinner and mentioned she'd seen me. Michelle asked, "Oh? What was she doing on the east coast?". Now, Mrs. Johnson had always liked me, as one of Sybil's friends. She made this clear in words when I was a teenager in Massachusetts, and later, in action, after I'd left for California. She would send me care packages of trinkets and gifts, just to let me know she was thinking of me. I always felt honored to be so accepted and cherished by a mom.

So, when Sybil brought up the incidents at Lawrence Academy, Mrs. Johnson told her she'd saved a few things. She went rifling through boxes. Soon, she produced a copy of the report Steve Hahn had typed up to the Department of Social Services, which she'd requested specifically in 1994. Documentation had been mysteriously lacking at present-day Lawrence Academy - so this was the first written record of events anyone had seen.

Michelle agreed to let Sybil send copies to me, to support my cause. Then, Mrs. Johnson told her daughter an additional story. She said she had always been disturbed by the lack of response by school administrators to this report and to Pete's actions. Sybil's father, Kevin, had always been quietly supportive behind the scenes, allowing Michelle to handle the interface of child, family, and school. Sybil had stayed on for the remainder of her high school years, and graduated in 1997, the same year as my sister.

The Johnson family still owed a balance of tuition to Lawrence Academy after their two children had graduated. Naturally, this was likely the case for most families at such a school. Well, Michelle got to the point where it just felt wrong paying them retroactively, given everything, and she decided to speak up about it.

In 2008, she wrote,

Lawrence Academy
Billing Department
Powderhouse Rd.
Groton, MA 01450

To Whom It May Concern,

A few years ago I wrote to the President of the school board requesting that all financial responsibilities, including loans, property liens, etc. by all members of the Johnson family be written off as a professional courtesy.

At that time it was referred back to the billing department, once again I am making this request not only for financial reasons but also due to the fact that although my children received a good education, the psychological impact of the incident involving Sybil makes it hard to deal with. It would be greatly appreciated if you would honor this request.

Sincerely,

Michelle Johnson

Sybil and I rejoiced at what this meant! First, it meant that Mrs. Johnson had taken a stand against the school's mishandling and found a way to gain restitution after the fact. Michelle told Sybil that Lawrence Academy simply stopped sending bills. That was almost a decade ago. It also served as verification of implied admission of guilt. A precedent had been set. Mrs. Johnson began searching for records to quantify how much the unofficial 'pardon' of debts had been worth. But, the real value lie in the gesture itself. She had essentially said, *"How about you just clear those books."*. As a mother myself at this point, I felt proud of her.

We had actual documents now - composed in Steve Hahn's words, which was intriguing in its own right - and the name of the employee who had received the report in 1994. We also had a hand-written note to Michelle Johnson. It read, with official letterhead on notepad paper:

STEVEN L. HAHN, Headmaster

LAWRENCE ACADEMY
Groton, Massachusetts 01450-0992
508-448-6535

August 17, 1994

Dear Michelle,

Enclosed is the copy of the DSS report. Please treat it confidentially. Let me know if you have any further concerns.

Sincerely,

Steve

"Please treat it confidentially", wrote the headmaster to the mother of a minor student who had been abused by school staff, in regards to the report she had to request to even see.

Fri, Mar 9, 2018, 4:57 PM

Dan,

I don't believe you are speaking truth. I don't think you believe, in good conscience, that the school is not responsible for what I endured, at least in the 10 years following my being excused after the abuse.

It is clear to me that you are now speaking on behalf of an institution - very carefully, as suggested by legal counsel. I am disappointed. The number, of course, is beyond insulting. More than that, I am disappointed to see that ultimately making things right was set aside for the sake of keeping the school comfortable.

Of course the school is liable for what happened. I know you know this.

I also find it unsettling to see that this offer is contingent upon confidentiality of terms and amounts. What is this? It almost reads like the school is - again - trying to cover this up as painlessly and quietly as possible. Does that small amount actually come with a contingency that I not speak about how the school (proposes it) handles this?

I am calling your bluff. This document is not honest.

I also wonder where you get your information, and how we could possibly have such differing ideas. I understand, by all counts, these kinds of cases yield at least the low six figures. I also have these resources [links to articles] to verify and give context to this.

I outline the story of Mrs. Johnson and clearing those books...

I am additionally confused about how you can admit wrongdoing (carefully, I notice, in your wording about "the school could have been more supportive"), while making pointed contingencies about not admitting legal liability.

How do you account for that discrepancy? What is the concern about admitting legal liability?

It seems to me you walk a continually thin line of invalidating your own words. I do want to believe you are capable of better, and higher.

. . . I sense you received some judgement early on about the number I proposed. (How did Mitchell Garabedian's number sit?, I wonder). I believe someone made a statement that allowed you to dismiss my claim as unreasonable and you have settled into the comfort of dismissing me as well.

I imagine you can deduce from our dealings so far — I will not be dismissed.

I later suggested to Dan Scheibe that Steve Hahn contribute to reaching a higher settlement amount. He commented that it was unlikely, but informed me that Steve was out of the country traveling, and he could coordinate a letter to such an effect. Steve's mailing address was intentionally kept from me. I did, however, have his cell phone number.

I left Steve Hahn a voicemail telling him I intended for him to contribute to reaching adequate settlement. I suggested that he give the equivalent to one year's salary in 1994. The way I saw it, I had demonstrated more leadership around the issue than he had. Like I'd said during my stay in Massachusetts, "It took me seven years to do what should have taken you five difficult minutes". At the end of my message, I briefly asked for permission to share his cell number with a few fellow alumni who also had concerns.

As I have often noticed, these modern information tools can just as readily be used as communication-avoidance tools. Steve Hahn texted me back in response.

Please do not share my cell phone number. Thank you for your concern.

Funny, he somehow missed the much larger concern about his accountability to this repair process. I said in response that I would honor his privacy when he honored my request. I replied,

What was your salary in 1994?

It was the first of many silences Steve Hahn then gave me along the way to forging a new path.

Diminishing - Stay Appropriate Size

After denial, the first thing many people-hiding-from-the-truth do is attempt to make the speaker-of-truth feel smaller. Really, they just want it to stop. The truth may be severely uncomfortable, and hearing it may cause them to shrink down within themselves in shame. So, if people-hiding-from-truth start collapsing inside, they may try to wound outwardly with the same weapon they are using internally.

Starting with compassion is always useful. Then, we must carry on with fierce determination.

The remedy for Diminishing is to Stay Appropriate Size. We do this by trusting our inner experience and defending it against making-you-small efforts. Confusing the reality or significance of a harmful act is one form of diminishing. Any message of, "Oh, that's just how it is," or "That's nothing, you're just making a big deal" tries to manipulate the scope of a situation. Remember, though; no one wrong-doer decides the significance of an event. Not even a group of well-paid wrong-doers. Wrong-doers don't get to decide the weight of what they have done. Two parties arrive at that truth by a joint effort of honest communication.

Stay Appropriate Size.

I responded to Dan Scheibe, "I have to say, the response from the school - this offer and letter you send - is hurtful and dismissive. It echoes of the exact response I received all along from the previous administration.

'This is not a big deal, take these minor consolations and walk away quietly now', is the message."

Go ahead and name it. Then, address the distortion and correct for errors.

I continue, "Your comment about my having a 'magnified view' of the impact struck me. I'll ask you to consider whether the inverse may be true. Perhaps, you have inherited a minimized view of what happened... as, clearly, many were invested in minimizing the story for obvious reasons."

Dan Scheibe was trying to make me and my experience small, in hopes of getting me to go away. Who has authority to name how "big" a wrong is? "*the money you are seeking is not commensurate with the wrongful conduct at issue*", wrote Bruce MacNeil. Who gets to say? Not the person who did it, nor the person who may be currently responsible.

If you stand up for yourself, and someone criticizes you, Diminishing may be at play. If they attack your character or something random like your clothing or body - see through this D tactic and commit to staying appropriate size. The person seeking to put you down is in a dark place. You need not follow.

Staying Appropriate Size means you don't puff up to counterattack - you don't back down and dismiss yourself or your perceptions. It means you keep firmly planted on a clear, high road. If I were to accept "Here's 3% now go away and don't tell anyone", or say to this school with a massive financial endowment, "No, I don't need money." I would have shrunk myself down too small. If I come at them with multiple lawyers, screaming my impacts and demanding millions, I would have gotten too big at the other extreme.

I conclude to Dan, "Beyond that, I know this is your world, and you love it, and it has served you well. I understand it is difficult to face the dark side of something that has sustained you and with which you identify. I do. That is the unpleasantness of my role here - I am insisting that this dark side be faced and acknowledged fully.

"Either way, I trust all will be revealed."

Go On, Tell Me to Be Quiet Again!

"If liberty means anything at all, it means
the right to tell people what they do not want to hear."

— George Orwell

For me, the voice of intuition speaks as insistent, almost nagging insights or ideas that return regularly over many days and give you positive energy for action.

First, let me say, I still fully believe in the power of Restorative Justice as a way through conflicts, harm, or interpersonal violations.

To state the obvious, agreeing to a certain time and then cancelling last-minute (especially on the harmed-party) is antithetical to the process. That move destroys trust. Every restorative practice must begin with the building of trust, setting agreements and creating a context that brings people to the table.

Secondly, no one gets to invalidate or "disagree" with anyone's lived experience before you even begin. They don't get to do that at any point. That move is also not restorative. In the Restorative Justice format, all voices are equal and given equitable time and consideration.

I was hurt that Dan Scheibe, Paul Lannon, and Steve Hahn demonstrated such extreme disrespect to the process, to me, and to

Saroeum's work. Their choices, I can't control. When people honor the process, though, Restorative Justice is profound in its ability to safely address harms and create healing in the wake of unfortunate incidents. I have been awed time and again by the power of this process done right.

I approached them with honesty, equality, and humanity; they met me with denial and diminishing. Yet, a truth never stays hidden for long.

Back at home in Washington, after the "here is what your suffering is worth" email exchange, this one idea circled back so often, it became hard to ignore. I imagined a short, animated video that told the story of a student returning year after year to the headmaster's office for right action following abuse. I could see little paper cut-outs of characters and the schoolhouse. I could hear the narration. After the video, there would be a petition people could sign, casting a vote on whether the school should settle with this student outside of court.

The title came to me, "The Amends Project, a Parable for Modern Times". It would be told in the style of a simple children's story. Even though I didn't use or understand social media, I appreciated its potential to spread a message, especially on issues people cared a lot about. In this moment in the United States' collective consciousness, there was a whole lot of care about how privileged men, in particular, were responding to allegations of abuse.

~ ~ ~

While #MeToo and TIMES UP movements stepped into light at the Oscars, and R Kelly concerts were being cancelled, as men in power positions were losing their jobs over allegations, I began making paper cut-outs. They would tell a story about abuse in boarding school culture and how pervasive cover-ups were in education. Soon, I realized I didn't have the skills to make a video or the extra time to acquire them (a more useful video would come later). So, I just started writing. I could do that.

I surprised myself by not wanting to put my name on the story initially. I just wanted the truth to be out, not to make it about me. I referenced a neutral "student" and focused on the patterns of secrecy in these schools. I created a petition, opened a new email address, and started a Wordpress website. It was just bare bones initially, with the story and the petition. But, it was a structure and a beginning. I sent the parable and the petition out by email to maybe 80-100 people I knew and considered allies. On May 8, 2018, The Amends Project website became a presence on the internet.

~~~

Then, I emailed every relevant person I could think of. I embarrassed myself with how many people I emailed. Hundreds. I followed threads of connection to the issue from alumni to trustees, parents, organization leaders, influential media people, and more. Old friends' names started appearing on the petition, and I followed up with a few of them.

With some momentum behind me now, it was time to contact all faculty and staff of current day Lawrence Academy.

Thu, May 3, 2018, 7:13 AM

The Amends Project - A Parable for Modern Times

Dear Concerned Member of the Lawrence Academy Community,

We ask you to take a moment to read the following story, which chronicles a current event in the movement toward justice for victims of child sexual abuse at Lawrence Academy.

If you read this tale, and are moved to action, we invite you to add your name to the petition, urging the school to complete the process of amends by full acknowledgement and settlement.

https://amendsproject.wufoo.com/forms/z1g2rfc60natzge/
~~~

If you know someone who may be affected by this story, feel free to forward it along. Thank you for your efforts to continually make Lawrence Academy a better place.

Kind Regards,

Vanessa, '96

Dan Scheibe caught wind of this story circulating around campus, and made a public statement which included his first, major ethical violation.

To the Lawrence Academy Community,

I am writing to you about a communication from a Lawrence Academy alumna that has been circulating within our community...

The case involved the actions of a former staff member, whom she identified as Pete Regis, a member of the facilities department. His actions involved [*here, Scheibe violates our Confidentiality Agreement by publicly disclosing details without my or Sybil's consent*] while working with female students in a shop area. According to our records, the school's leadership was notified at the time, health services were offered to the student, and her parents were notified. In addition, the employee was removed from campus housing [*Pete Regis' wife divorced him a few years after we confronted him about the abuse. The school kept Regis in his same position - but his wife soon told him to move out*] and forbidden from having any further direct contact with students. In keeping with our legal obligation and with sound practice, the school informed the state agency overseeing child welfare at the time the incident was reported [*yet, not the police, which is a violation of both school policy and "legal obligation"*]. That agency decided not to open an investigation based on the allegations.

... Sadly, we cannot change the events or acts of the past [*has anyone asked for this?*]. However, in the present day of Lawrence Academy, we have consistently taken action to ensure our campus is a safe environment in which students can thrive with a sense of protection and security. On behalf of the school, we firmly pledge to maintain this resolve of care.

Sincerely,

Dan Scheibe
Head of School

What does it mean, when Dan Scheibe says "That agency decided not to open an investigation based on the allegations."? What is he saying? Was that decision truly based on the allegations, or was some other factor involved in the failure to investigate?

Is he implying something about the severity of incidents or about where responsibility for ethical response actually lies?

From the documents surfaced by the Johnson family, I now had the name of the woman who'd taken the report in 1994: Marcia Graves. I did a search for Marcia Graves (Roddy) and found an article which described failure to follow through on reports of abuse, at what is now called the Massachusetts Department of Children and Families.

Worcester Telegram
August 29, 2015

Lawsuit alleges DCF staff lied to police in Oliver case[5]

---

5 Paula Owen, The Worcester Telegram, August 25. 2015, https://www.telegram.com/article/20150829/NEWS/150829132

A lawsuit filed in Worcester Superior Court by a social worker who used to work in the state Department of Children and Families office in Leominster, during the time staff there was charged with providing services to Jeremiah Oliver's family, alleges supervisors and managers did not follow through with reviews on numerous high-risk cases and allegedly lied to investigators in the Jeremiah Oliver case.

Many feel Jeremiah was failed by DCF when a social worker in the Leominster office skipped eight mandatory monthly visits with the 5-year-old Fitchburg boy, who *[died a horrible death sometime in 2013-14 - I choose to not repeat those details here]*

The case led to the firing of his social worker and two of her supervisors.

The cases have placed DCF under heavy public scrutiny and have people asking why the state's top child welfare agency cannot do better by the children it is supposed to protect.

In former social worker Sara A. Vasquez's lawsuit filed Aug. 18 in Worcester Superior Court, she alleges supervisors and managers in the Leominster office should have done more with cases involving multiple reports of abuse and neglect. She alleges she was fired, in part, in retaliation for complaints she made about the handling of the Oliver case. She is seeking $725,000 in damages - $375,000 for past and future lost wages and $350,000 for injuries.

The defendants named in the case are: DCF; the Commonwealth of Massachusetts; the Executive Office of Health and Human Services; Lian Hogan, acting interim regional director overseeing DCF's central and western regions at the time of the Oliver case; and **Marcia Graves Roddy**, area director for DCF's north and south central offices during the Oliver case. Mr. Hogan was Ms. Roddy's superior and both oversaw North Central area managers Jacque Carl and David Rondeau and the social worker and supervisors who were fired.

What does it mean if a state agency does not open an investigation into a report of abuse? Simply put: someone didn't do their job.

~ ~ ~

Once I saw this public statement, I immediately called Dan Scheibe and yelled at him for breaking confidentiality. *"How could you feel entitled to spread those details without my consent?! We had a legally binding agreement!"*. He blundered and attempted defensiveness. But, the online version of the statement then had the details omitted; all evidence was quickly removed. It was yet another violation that would have stood had I not discovered it and spoken out. I remember this moment well because it took me a full three hours of vigorous hiking with the dog to process the level of RAGE over their decision.

In addition to the phone call, I sent an email.

May 22, 2018, 9:07 AM

to dscheibe

You recognize this is a very big deal, yes? Not only did disclosing personal details violate decency and trust - it was also a violation of our Confidentiality Agreement for the Restorative Justice Circle.

It reads, "The Parties are disclosing sensitive and confidential information in reliance upon this Agreement, and any breach of this Agreement would cause irreparable injury for which monetary damages would be inadequate. Consequently, any Party to this Agreement may obtain an injunction to prevent disclosure of any such confidential information in violation of this Agreement."

Guidelines put forth by the School Counselors Association regarding the handling of sexual abuse details state: "The need-to-know rule requires school counselors reveal sensitive information only when the recipients of the information has a need to know *and is in a position to benefit the student* if they have the shared information."

Clearly, you have done this for MY benefit, yes?

~ ~ ~

Then, after casting my story into the vast unknown over email, I got a call one night from reporter Rick Sobey at The Lowell Sun. The call came around 8 pm, which meant it was nearly 11 pm on the east coast when he called. His voice was earnest, and he spoke slowly. "I got your email...". There was a stunned, in-the-moment processing sense about it. "This is like the stories from The Boston Globe's Spotlight investigation..." He asked if we could make an appointment to do an interview. I agreed. I chose a time when I had a few hours of free time two days later. I knew a door was now opening.

Rick and I got on the phone, and I told him all that I had, from the very beginning. He took notes and asked only a few questions. But mostly, I just relived it. He said, "Wow" a lot, and we rolled through the details. Once we got to present-tense, we paused, and Rick said, "We've been talking for two and a half hours, and it feels like we've been on the phone for twenty minutes."

Then came the issue of using my name. I wasn't fully convinced yet, so we talked about the choice. As a reporter, he said the story would be much more powerful with a name attached. I told him I'd consider it, as long as he agreed to include my petition. The point of my outreach was to influence a new outcome, where leaders would admit to their cover-up behavior and de-normalize the practice. It would give people an outlet for their outrage with action. He said yes, he would include it. I agreed to put my name on the story.

There was just a little correspondence back and forth over the following days. I remember Sobey said, "We just have to make sure we don't get sued by the school.". I sent pictures, and the Lowell Sun team confirmed details. Then, it was all ready.

Being on a nation-wide podcast stretched my comfort edge on exposure. This step sent me over that edge. My whole body was jumpy and heightened, leading up to release. I was constantly pacing and shaking out my limbs to calm myself. Still, I was resolute. I understood that these kinds of power abuses thrive in silence - so the antidote was to speak the truth of what happened at Lawrence Academy. I'd given so much of my life to making things right already. I decided my ego could recede into the larger purpose. What is this life, if not put to use in service of something greater?

I could barely physically tolerate reading it when he sent the link. I was on system overload. I felt put off by the title right away, and the sensational opening. But, I relaxed some as I read the balance of points throughout...

The Feature Article, The Lowell Sun

A NIGHTMARE WITHOUT END[6]

By **RICK SOBEY**
PUBLISHED: May 26, 2018 at 12:00 a.m. | UPDATED: July 11, 2019 at 12:00 a.m.

GROTON — Vanessa Fadjo peered out her dorm window — trembling, stomach churning.

A man who had allegedly sexually molested her stood in the front yard, staring up at her window.

The 14-year-old at Lawrence Academy in Groton was terrified to leave her dorm. The 39-year-old employee still roamed the campus.

She approached the headmaster several times, pleading with the school leader to remove the alleged child molester.

Year after year, she was told it would be handled, but never was.

"They knew something was wrong and kept choosing to do nothing about it," she told The Sun last week. She's now 40 and has the last name Osage.

---

6 Rick Sobey, The Lowell Sun, May 27, 2018, https://theamendsproject.com/press/

In a statement to The Sun last week, current Head of School Dan Scheibe wrote, "Had the same set of circumstances presented themselves today, there is no question that we would have immediately terminated the staff member from employment at the school."

. . . It is fair to say, however, that the school is not in full agreement with several of the alumna's claims and statements."

Attempts to reach Regis were unsuccessful. His last known address is in Windsor, South Carolina, and the phone number listed did not go to voicemail; the line wouldn't stop ringing. His two Groton home addresses listed expired in 1995 and 1999, respectively. He's 65 today.

. . . The state agency did not open an investigation based on the allegations, Scheibe said in a statement. In addition, Scheibe said the employee was removed from campus housing and forbidden from having further direct contact with students.
Regis remained exactly where he was on campus, Osage stressed. Within a week of the meeting, Osage said, Regis started stalking her at her dorm.

Osage went to Hahn, asking what would be done. Hahn, she said, told her that Regis had been placed on a kind of suspension contract.

"'If he does it again, he'll have to go,'" Osage recalled Hahn saying.

"I was blown away by him wanting to take that risk. Just stunned," she said. Hahn, reached by The Sun, referred to the school's statement to The Sun, and declined to comment further.

FINANCIAL AID

Before her junior year, she says the school revoked her financial aid but not her sister's.

"It was the easiest cover-up option they had," said Osage, who transferred to Acton-Boxboro Regional High School.

Scheibe said the school did not, and would never, withhold financial aid as a retaliatory measure. He added the school cannot comment on any one case because financial support is confidential.

. . . In front of a full auditorium in December 2001, Osage told her story about Regis, and about the school's response. She wanted to help the students stay safe, guide them to know about their body, and pay attention to what feels right to them.

Regis, employed for seven years after the documented abuse, was let go on permanent long-term disability in 2001, she said.

"The heartbreak for me is that my health was slowly going downhill, but they made sure his health was taken care of," Osage said.

. . . Osage hired a lawyer who sent a letter to the school demanding a $2 million settlement. The lawyer, however, wasn't open to a restorative justice approach, in which the school acknowledges the facts about the school's handling of abuse. That was key for Osage. As a result, she went on her own.

She calculated that her losses and damages was $640,000 — mental-health expenses, surgery expenses, loss of work, travel expenses and more.

. . . In addition, Scheibe wrote that [former headmaster Steve] Hahn "respectfully declines" her request for him to acknowledge liability.

Osage said over and over in her interviews with The Sun that she will not accept those terms.

"I won't let this go," she said. "I have devoted so much of my life to this. I am committed to doing this thoroughly and in an ethical way."

Her hope is that before graduation on Friday, June 1, the school will acknowledge the facts of the school's handling and will reach her minimum settlement without a confidentiality clause.

"I'm presenting them with an opportunity to rise to being a role model on how to resolve these situations," she said.

"Transformation is still possible."

~ ~ ~

My heart rattled my whole body as I tried to use my eyes to focus on these words and continue breathing. Yet, I felt like a freight train speeding along this risky ride, until I hit the stone mountain. **He did not include the petition**. The words The Amends Project were completely absent, as was any reference to my current professional work. I shook in slow rhythm with my own rapid-beating heart and felt stunned.

Then, I was immediately calling Rick Sobey.

"Rick, you promised me you would include my petition!", I exhaled, trying to contain my panic and my rage. "Oh, right, I probably should have emailed you...". His soft, distanced tone was its own devastation. "The Editor decided last-minute to take it out, so it didn't look like we were taking sides.".

"But, I had your word", I countered, part rage, part tears now. "I know", he said. "I'm sorry".

I continued, "Now people are going to have no way to take action on this - nothing to do with all the energy they feel. It's such a waste..." He feigned understanding, from behind the safety of his position - and the inevitability of the story already having gone to print. Drivers were delivering this feature article all over the Lowell/Boston area as we spoke.

I got off the phone and walked outside. I raged. I broke things. Yet another man had lied, taken liberties that were not his - going against his own word - and stolen some personal advantage. It was fucking terrible. "It's not entertainment", I fumed. "It's a call to action!".

I'd made a big step, but with the potent reminder of how pervasive this disease of 'male privilege' was at every turn. The story was out. It was sensationalist, but balanced. The breaking of silence was like breaking out of my parents' home by running through the plate-glass door. All points of contact breaking in one disastrous glass shower around me. I could only hope these would be small scratches on my arm as I covered vast, new ground next.

Still, They Came - Waking Up

Of course, find me they did. I had no idea how powerful that urge would be - for people to connect with someone who was speaking the truth they had been bullied into silently holding.

Old classmates, and total strangers, took the risk to send messages to my organization email at Rooted Emerging. This was the first email contact that came up when you searched my name back then. I first discovered all of these people who'd known me in high school and wondered what happened to me. They were lovingly relieved to see me surface again. Then, there were those holding a similar pain. I imagine what they had to overcome in themselves, the doubts and reservations, to share private information they could only hope would reach me. With more and more frequency, they did.

The petition signers grew, and I was able to map where in the world people had viewed the small website. Similar stories were echoing:

"Thank you for your courage in speaking out and not letting anyone try to buy your silence. I attended Lawrence from 1990 to 1992. During the 1991-1992 school year a teacher told me that that he felt there had been a cover up by administration after a student spoke to the school staff about alleged sexual assault by a peer. Transparency and accountability is needed."

Along with support:

"I remember hearing a similar story about Mr. Regis and a young girl (it was my senior year). I have no doubt that this story is true. I hope that LA starts taking responsibility for what happened to these women, and in the future, makes it a priority to protect their students who are brave enough to come forward with stories of sexual harassment or abuse. I hope Vanessa gets everything she needs to move on."

~ ~ ~

Once I made peace with what I could no longer change - that while confronting patriarchy, I was going to meet the ills of patriarchy - I realized I now had options. I could do something with this. Time to move forward.

First, I wrote most of what would be an article and asked Rick to incorporate it into a follow-up piece. The title, "Nightmare Without End" had disturbed me because it implied futility. This situation was absolutely not futile. I was on a path to ending this trend. Running with that imagery, I thought, '*well, nightmares end when we wake up.*'. So, I organized a positive action, asking people to simply wear yellow to graduation, to symbolize the rising sun and their support of resolution in The Amends Project.

I sent the draft to Rick, who soon responded with, "The Editor thinks it's a better fit for an editorial.". Right.

So, I wrote one:

Former Student Urges Lawrence Academy, "Wake Up!"

In an ongoing effort for reconciliation of mishandling of child sexual abuse, former student Vanessa (Fadjo) Osage is calling on the surrounding community to attend graduation on Friday June 1, wearing yellow.

The yellow is meant to represent the rising sun, and an end to the darkness of covering up crimes against children, especially at our most prestigious institutions: a simple, non-threatening action.

The name of the effort is a response to Sunday's feature article by Rick Sobey, "A Nightmare Without End". Vanessa Osage, of Love & Truth Rising, says, "This needs to end the way all nightmares end - we wake up".

The wake up Osage is calling for includes two steps: Accountability & Reparation. So far, the current administration has been willing to acknowledge the actions of the alleged child molester, but continues to deny any wrong-doing on the part of the school's leaders.

The move is the latest in a long string of actions - first for her own protection as a student - and later, for the safety of students after her. Letters, visits, a speech to expose the school, and most recently, an online petition with educational website (www.theamendsproject.com).

Then, I emailed the faculty and staff of Lawrence Academy again, knowing they'd seen or heard about the feature article. I included the local police, nearby organizations, and more.

May 30, 2018 9:36 AM

Faculty, Staff & the Surrounding Lawrence Academy Community,

As you all start preparing to celebrate on Friday, I need to remind you that a large, unresolved issue lingers in the hearts and minds of people all around the region and the world...

I need you all to see it for what it is: a shameful tale of an institution placing its reputation above the well-being of its students at great expense, for many, many years. You cannot change the past - but you all can absolutely be a part of creating a more positive future for Lawrence Academy today.

This would be worth celebrating.

I ask you all, as I have asked hundreds/thousands in the region - wake up from this nightmare and call a stop to it. Wear yellow on graduation day and say that you want a time when all students are seen, believed, protected and honored...

Earnestly,

Vanessa (Fadjo) Osage, '96

~ ~ ~

Rick Sobey owed me one. So, I wrote:

Wed, May 30, 2018, 5:42 AM

Rick,

I wake up still feeling torn up about the article coming out without any reference to my efforts (the website/petition) as promised.

I agreed to share my name as long as my wishes were respected and I was consulted.

So, I am asking for your help...

Please sign the petition and share it with all of your circles. Please attend the graduation on Friday as a reporter, wearing yellow, and bring as many people as you can.

I have come a very long way, against great odds and this deserves to be met with similar good efforts by those who come into contact with it.

Please let me know.

Thank You,

Vanessa

Wed, May 30, 2018, 8:41 AM

Hi Vanessa,

I totally understand where you are coming from on this.

I hope to attend graduation on Friday at Lawrence Academy as a reporter.

Have a great day,
Rick

Friday June 1, 2018 came and went and I heard nothing. Finally, Rick checked in.

Jun 4, 2018, 5:51 AM

Hi Vanessa,

Yes, I was turned away from graduation on Friday. I couldn't believe it. I hadn't even introduced myself, and they came over to me, kicking me off campus.

Here is the editorial in today's paper.

Have a great day,
Rick

EDITORIAL: Lawrence Academy bans the media[7]

[7] Jim Campinini, The Lowell Sun, June 4, 2018, https://theamendsproject.com/press/

By **LOWELL SUN**
PUBLISHED: June 4, 2018 at 12:00 a.m. I UPDATED: July 11, 2019 at 12:00 a.m.

Lawrence Academy, a private boarding school in Groton, set a new standard of elitist exclusivity Friday night: It kicked off its campus a journalist assigned to cover the school's graduation ceremony.
The reporter, Rick Sobey, works for this media organization, which includes The Sun of Lowell, Sentinel and Enterprise of Fitchburg, and the Nashoba Valley Voice.

On Friday, the newspapers covered 10 high school graduations from Lowell to Lunenburg without a hitch, except for Lawrence Academy.
Head of School Dan Scheibe declined to issue a statement for Lawrence Academy's action.

But we believe we have the reason.

It was in retaliation for an article Sobey wrote titled "A Nightmare Without End". Published Sunday, May 27, it told the story of Vanessa Fadjo Osage, now 40, who, as a Lawrence Academy junior [*freshman, as a correction*] in 1993, was sexually molested by a school groundskeeper. Osage was 14 at the time.

Despite knowledge of the employee's actions, school officials allowed the man, then 39, to remain in his job for seven years until he was finally let go. Osage said she wasn't the only victim, and for years she's struggled emotionally over the school's mishandling of the allegations.

Osage told Sobey she went public because she was frustrated over settlement negotiations with present-day Lawrence Academy officials.

Initially, the school had asked people to come forward if they had information about past or current sexual misconduct. Osage obliged with documents showing school officials knew of her molestation claims against the groundskeeper, identified as Peter Regis. She said the school protected

Regis — he kept his job — and retaliated against her — Osage's financial aid package was revoked.

. . . There's no doubt that a former Lawrence Academy administration conducted an egregious coverup and that present-day officials are trying to make amends. While the latter is laudable, the new regime seems reluctant to embrace transparency and accept responsibility for the sins of the past.

In 1993, Vanessa Fadjo Osage was robbed of her teen-age innocence at Lawrence Academy and school officials rejected her to avoid a scandal about a child molester on campus.

On Friday, the school retaliated against the newspaper that told Osage's compelling story.

It's clear Lawrence Academy officials still can't handle the truth about what happened 26 years ago.

Tue, Jun 5, 2018, 1:32 PM

Hi Vanessa,

It was a bizarre situation there last Friday. I was happy my editor wrote this editorial.

I would recommend you follow-up writing to my editors with the Letter to the Editor with your website, cc'ing me as well.

I hope they publish it for you.

Have a great day!
Rick

OPINION I EDITORIALS

Lawrence Academy sex-abuse victim says she won't be a silent accomplice[8]

By **LOWELL SUN**
PUBLISHED: June 10, 2018 at 12:00 a.m. I UPDATED: July 11, 2019 at 12:00 a.m.

I write today with a mix of relief, frustration and concern. My name is Vanessa Osage and I am the former student seeking amends from Lawrence Academy. First, I thank you for your attention to this story. As a sexuality educator, consultant/coach and leader of a mission-driven business, I care about this today for a number of reasons.

First, we must understand that sexual abuse and/or harassment do not happen in a vacuum. They are perpetrated by abusers, bystanders and enablers. When someone turns away or supports institutions that allow abuse, these players are also accountable. In this story, I suggest the key players are even more accountable than a man who was ill and acting out.

I have been asked by Lawrence Academy on numerous occasions over the course of decades to be a silent accomplice to these crimes. I will not. Not when they send me away, not when they attempt to control my message, not when they offer pocket change amends, but only if I am quiet about it.

I speak now, as I did then, because the bigger picture of these abuses matters. How every one of us responds to these issues matters. I have created a website where you may direct your energy into action: www.theamendsproject.com

---

8 Vanessa Osage, The Lowell Sun, June 10, 2018, https://theamendsproject.com/press/

We Are With You

"However much you deny the truth,
the truth goes on existing."

— George Orwell

In June, this email came from Rick Sobey:

Hi Vanessa,

This information was sent to me today. Do you have any idea about this? Please keep this between you and me.

Thanks,
Rick

He attached an excerpt of a scanned, typed letter, sent to The Lowell Sun by mail with no return address:

"Further, they represent another example of the silencing of bad behavior by the people responsible for protecting our children.

Eric Peterson is the brother-in-law of Dan Scheibe, head of school at Lawrence Academy in Groton, MA. Eric Peterson's wife (Krista) is the sister of Dan Scheibe's wife (Annie Montesano).

Eric Peterson's son, xxxx Peterson, was a student at Lawrence Academy as a sophomore (unknown where he attended his freshman year or why he left there) and for a short time as a junior. During xxxx's sophomore year at Lawrence Academy he is alleged to have assaulted a female student. It was not reported to the police and he remained a student at the school. At the beginning of his junior year (Fall of 2014) he allegedly assaulted a second female student. This time he was dismissed from Lawrence Academy.

The two girls xxxx is alleged to have assaulted are both currently seniors at Lawrence Academy. It is rumored that both girl's families were convinced not to press charges and were compensated for their silence. Some maintain that their tuition was waived. Many in the Lawrence Academy community know about both incidents. Most students know the identity of both of xxxx's victims.

xxxx Peterson is now attending the Canterbury School, a private boarding school in New Milford, CT. My guess is few if any of those students know about xxxx's past, leaving yet another set of students vulnerable to his behavior."

There it was. Confirmation that the larger problem of secrecy and silencing had, in alleged fact, survived to the modern day. If this were true, then things were clearly NOT better now. They were acting like people with something to hide, and I had found the reason why. More accurately, it had found me.

One petition-signer wrote this in 2018:

"I went to Lawrence Academy and witnessed cover ups of sexual assaults and many other horrific things. This is just the beginning. Scheibe, we're coming for you."

Sybil and I talked, to connect about this discovery. Cover-ups were, allegedly, still happening at Lawrence Academy of Groton, Massachusetts. It was heart-wrenching. Since we'd walked the long road already together, we could easily look far into the future together, as well. She said, "Kids need somewhere they can go at school when something happens - somewhere that's not a Steve Hahn or a Dan Scheibe, but a diverse group of people to choose from... a person of color, an LGBTQ person, more women than men..."

I said, "They need somewhere to go *outside* the school, so something can actually be done about it.".

I soaked up her steady wisdom and strong heart a while longer, and we hung up the phone. Then, I sat in a long silence, thinking about all the seeming progress we'd made, and remembering my intention with The Amends Project.

I did some research and browsed the Reporting Policies for Lawrence Academy. It read,

"Once a report is received from Ethics Point [the current communication system], the school determines whether to investigate the matter internally, or whether an external entity (such as law enforcement or an outside consultant) should be brought in."

There it was. The cover-up loophole!

According to this language, the school could determine whether to "handle it" internally or to involve outside officials. Right! They had simply determined - in the 1990s as in the 2010s - to handle it internally. This language even suggested that school officials could decide to not bring in law enforcement, if it best suited them. It was written right into their policies.

It's funny what will lull people into complacency, a few reassuring words here, a few boastful public statements there.

A family might browse these policies and miss the stipulation or the larger implications. *'Oh, right, they'll figure out how to best handle it.'*. Only, that gives headmasters, trustees, and attorneys disproportionate power to make their own call about whether or not something is serious. They decide whether the person who abused a student will be expelled (more likely if they are a minority, or of African-American descent) or let go without consequence (say, if your family was on the Board or in the headmaster's chair).

It says it right there.

Of course, that information could just as easily be redirected outside the school to people who would make that determination, free from racial, gender, socioeconomic bias, or nepotism. Outside the school was where those decisions needed to be made, in full, ethical collaboration with families - where they have nothing to fear or to lose.

On an afternoon in July, I sketched out a plan for an oversight and transparency model. This was what I wanted, as part of my ultimate settlement with Lawrence Academy. Eight weeks after going public with the website, I proposed this model, The Justice CORPS - the Committee to Oversee Rights & Protections of Students - to Dan Scheibe and Paul Lannon as part of my resolution.

They immediately declined.

~ ~ ~

Still, I wanted the kids watching all of this - the current students - to know there was an older generation of former students seeing the problem and working on it. I emailed Rick Sobey to ask if he'd been able to confirm the anonymous tip. He had not. He referred to the challenge of confidentiality agreements around it. I told him it was time for me to reference it. I promised I would not mention his name, nor would I mention the Lowell Sun. Then, I redacted the names and posted it on The Amends Project website, with the words: We Are With You.

Falling & Rising

"Societies in decline have no use for visionaries."

— Anais Nin

Miraculous or shocking things seemed to surface every few days now. So, one day I got an email from an old family friend. He'd been a classmate at Lawrence Academy, too. Just seeing his name brought a big, familiar smile. He and my sister had dated, our parents were connected. Alex Hayes walked in the world with the kind of golden heart you'd want in any neighborhood boy. Now, he was a grown man with an education in law. The title of his email read, "Wow—" and opened with:

"I always thought you were pretty amazing, but now I know for sure..."

He wanted me to see what he'd posted on Facebook. It read:

I recently found out that my high school produced a woman who did the hardest thing in the world. I encourage you to read this article, read my opinion, and keep the conversation moving... *[link to June 4, 2018 editorial by Lowell Sun Editor Jim Campinini "Lawrence Academy Bans the Media"]*

Today, LA is faced with a dilemma that will cement its own legacy and I deeply trust that continued discourse and publication can influence the correct course of action. The question for the court of public opinion is one that has been asked by at least one former student for years yet lacks a properly balanced reply.

Lawrence admin; how do you move forward when faced with the news that a faculty member was doing the type of thing that adult males do in situations of power and trust? To be clear; crossing a deeply personal, adolescent boundary without consent. Tough question at first, I'm sure. Let's take a look at your efforts and construct a fair evaluation. Initially, it appears that your response was to push away the hand of the student when she came to you for help. If that's true, if you turned away a victim to shoulder YOUR problem by herself, that's an abject failure of your fiduciary duty to your consumers and to the public. Let's assume its also true that she continued to return for answers, year after year, and that you continued to relentlessly push her away. It appears you chose the hand of the accused every time and danced with him instead, in silence for years. If this is true I am in awe of the true power of elitism and its ability to dehumanize the faces I trusted on that campus. It's fascinating really. In fairness, this is an accounting by a brave victim and numerous publications in the media - I would objectively evaluate a counter statement if I were to see one. Problem is, I don't...

An objective evaluation of the statements made by the victim, the dilatory timing of the confirmation, the fiduciary responsibility involved, leads to a conclusion that accountability is an issue here. But it's a layered issue. For instance, if money weren't involved, I am beyond confident that you would have done the right thing, as if she was your own child, but protecting the shield was a priority and if true, despite your responsibility to do the right thing, money muted your morality. That is something YOU have to live with, forever, alone.

We all agree in theory, that children of the families who pay you are more important than the money they give you. Pretty simple. I hope LA can turn "Me too" in to an opportunity to help someone. It doesn't look like they truly have yet...so I encourage LA to embrace this opportunity and choose the right mold for their future (it's not hush payments). I hope they can remove the appearance of corruption that goes with well-financed education like ivy goes with brick. Until then I wonder how parents will evaluate a tuition of around $50k. $60k if they live on campus (yikes!).

Friends, you have a chance to be part of progress, please consider signing this petition. The link below provides a narrative and a place to find updates. We are all setting examples for our children by our decisions. Vanessa is an example I will be sharing with my daughters.

As Alex lifted the conversation to this level, people of similar conscience chimed in - and soon, I gained a highly valuable advisor. Noah Elder added this to the petition:

"I remember meeting Vanessa the first day of freshman orientation for Lawrence Academy class of 1996. Vanessa was bright, charismatic, and radiant. The orientation was the introduction not only to new classmates but the establishment of community. The school made many lofty goals for the community at the interlocken wilderness. Community is a lofty ideal for high schoolers and yet somehow we all did our part. Learning that a predator was knowingly allowed to stay within our community is devastating. I admire Vanessa's endurance, determination, and strength. I commend Vanessa's valiant service to the community in standing up, persisting, and ridding Lawrence Academy of a predator. Thank you Vanessa for speaking out and rallying your community. We were promised better and with your efforts may we be better."

Noah, like Alex, was a hugely positive association for me. We hadn't been close friends or in the same friend-groups in high school. Yet, we shared a mutual respect that transcended social stratification as teenagers. We always seemed to understand each other. So, to see his name and words all these years later was an incredible blessing.

I followed up with a phone call, and we connected for the first time in well over twenty years. Noah had also studied law and referred to himself at this stage as an "entrepreneurial attorney". Among his many innate gifts was this remarkable ability to know the world of the elites and also to witness their inner working from a place of wise insightfulness. He was in that world, but not of it. His perspectives were like gold, every one of them.

~ ~ ~

It was time for me to address the xxxx Peterson incidents with headmaster Dan Scheibe. I invited him to a video conference to discuss The Justice CORPS proposal. He agreed. On July 22, 2018, we got everything set up, and started in to talking again, in digital view of one another. His camera was angled in such a way that I saw a 45-degree angle of his face. He looked to a corner (where he saw my image), and I looked directly into the camera, at a slanted view of him. This angle accentuated what came next.

He initially seemed light and unattached, in a classic stance of 'innocence' around all of this. To my perception, Scheibe still clung to some relief at the thought that the focus was mostly on players of the past. Even any question I might ask, about my current settlement, carried this air. He could defer to a mysteriously-hidden set of decision-makers. Or, if that failed, he could direct me to attorney Paul Lannon. The web of complacency traces the same lines as the maze of dodging accountability. Scheibe seemed to believe that nowhere was *he* actually on the line in any of this. Of course, now I knew otherwise.

About twenty minutes in, I changed the subject. "Also, Dan, I need to talk to you about a new issue." He clenched up some. I said, "I know about the xxxx Peterson incidents.". Then, he visibly twitched and spasmed all through his body. I asked, "Is that true?". He countered, as if rehearsing lines from that same old marionette-play I'd witnessed back in March, "We are aware of this, and if you have any concerns, you can talk to Paul Lannon about it.".

I let the absurdity of his response hang in the air a moment. Then, I laughed in an exhale of obvious disgust, "Of course I have concerns!".

Paul, of course, ignored all of my questions about the incidents. No response at all. Still, I had all the confirmation I needed.

~ ~ ~

An alumna and dear old friend had become very vocal and started spreading the petition to friends around the world. I had great love for her as a friend. She was bright, warm-hearted, free-spirited, and open with love for the world. We had met my senior year and reconnected once on the west coast after I ran away. She asked in a fury, "What can I do? I'm good at rallying the troops...". She'd added to the online petition:

"I was a student at Lawrence Academy the same time Vanessa was there and am appalled and deeply saddened to hear what occurred during this time. I know Vanessa to be one of the most honest, humble, gentle and kind people I have ever met and if she says this happened, I believe her 150% as should you all. As a mother of a young girl myself, I am even more disgusted as I know how vulnerable our young children are in the hands of supposed trusted adults, especially those who slowly creep their way in to push boundaries and violate trust. I would hope that if this had been my daughter or me that anyone and everyone would have stood up and fought to make sure I was protected, not silenced. I am so sad she had to endure this alone. I also have no doubt this would have happened to a large number of other students at LA during those years as Peter Regis was well known for having one on one time with students in his workshop on a regular basis. It is absolutely horrific to imagine that he was not immediately fired and handed over to the police and that he continued being employed there for seven years after this occurred. I hope the school and administration past and present will do the right thing and take full responsibility for not protecting Vanessa and other students from this predator and help make amends in any and every way possible."

She was from Los Angeles, California, and had connections in the entertainment industry. She started reaching out to reporters, celebrities, and soon - she suggested I consider going on the Ellen Show.

Remembering the intensity I had to manage while the feature article came out, I took a moment. Television?! I hadn't even watched television since 1998. I told her I'd have to sleep on it.

I again arrived at the same conclusion, about allowing my ego to be absorbed into a larger purpose. It would absolutely terrify me, and maybe help me grow. Bigger results ask for bigger steps. I became willing. I wrote back to say, yes, I would do it. She responded, "You are a goddess. You are absolutely saving lives.".

~ ~ ~

Days later, I sent my new settlement terms to Dan, Paul, and Board of Trustees President, Bruce MacNeil. I hadn't met Bruce, but he had been there during my time in the 1990s, and his name showed up at the end of public statements. All of the actual "decision-makers" had been intentionally kept from me. Now, I was starting to sense he was one of the main puppet masters.

I laid out my new terms:

1. A draft of a public statement, crafted jointly by Steven L Hahn & R Daniel Scheibe to acknowledge the cover-up of sending me away, disallowing return for my junior year, following the incidents with Peter Regis. Acknowledging the problem of secrecy that has harmed students, in the wake of problems that have arisen.

2. Written confirmation of $500,000 settlement, as personal injury.

3. Agreement to participate in a pilot program of the Justice CORPS, outlined below, starting in the 2018-2019 school year.

4. Finally, in anticipation of my having a national television platform - as soon as this week - I encourage the following steps be taken, in regards to xxxx Peterson:

Informing Canterbury Academy in writing about xxxx's history, by September 1, 2018, to headmaster, assistant headmaster, and all seven members of their health team (9 letters): [link to their contacts]

5. Ensure that xxxx is enrolled in three continuous months of perpetrator treatment counseling by September 1, 2018:

[link to a local therapist specializing in perpetrator treatment]

My recommendation is to arrange for treatment and to include a letter from his counselor to each of the school faculty. With this addressed, I will not feel the need to share this story any further.

From Bruce MacNeil, in response:

"...the board cannot accept your proposal as we still disagree with some of your conclusions."

I asked repeatedly for clarification on this "disagreement". I got long-winded, superfluous language that dodged the point. So, I later asked again:

Dan, Bruce,

Please define the disagreement as you see it, in three sentences or less. What claims are you disagreeing with? Be specific.

Nothing.

~ ~ ~

Then, another former student who'd had similar experiences with Pete Regis came forward. She was choosing to sue. I felt terrified to consider it could have been someone younger than myself - my most immense fear from 1994-2001. I contacted Bruce MacNeil to ask what year she attended, and he evaded my question. I finally learned from a classmate of hers that she'd been there a few years before I had. Relief. There I was, 25 years later, rattled over whether school leaders' decisions had allowed a preventable abuse on campus. I was still panic-stricken by it. This friend of the woman who came forward had signed my petition and gave me the relief and clarification I needed: this former student suing came before.

Now, in addition to my new, alternate efforts, a former student was filing a law suit against Lawrence Academy. Dan Scheibe and Bruce MacNeil put their names on a new, public statement. They announced an investigation with Sanghavi Law Office, and concluded:

...The circumstances leading to this investigation are painful to reckon with. Nevertheless, we must learn as much as we can about what happened in our past so that we can face matters squarely today and move forward proactively in the interests of all of our students.

Sincerely,

Dan Scheibe, Head of School
Bruce MacNeil, President of the Board of Trustees

That last line read, again, "so that we can face matters squarely today and move forward proactively in the interests of all of our students." *In the interests of all of our students*. Please also note a marked change in tone, since the statement about my coming forward. The matter of Pete Regis' behavior was serious, it read. The matter of school leaders' choice to keep him employed and living among students while I pleaded for right action? A lost cause, and an issue in the past, they suggested. This statement again, from May:

"… Sadly, we cannot change the events or acts of the past. However, in the present day of Lawrence Academy, we have consistently taken action to ensure our campus is a safe environment in which students can thrive with a sense of protection and security. On behalf of the school, we firmly pledge to maintain this resolve of care."

Sincerely,

Dan Scheibe
Head of School

A Breather for Healing

One night, amidst a frenzy of messages from people I'd never met, while corresponding with The Lowell Sun to get my latest Editorial into print, a strange feeling came over me. It was after midnight. I was alone in a big house, emailing well after my healthy cut-off time. I was over-alert and a bit jumpy. Sure, my heart was racing as I felt the pressure of trying to represent a mix of people in various degrees of pain, while exposing myself to the media in a way that still felt foreign. It was too much. I felt exhausted but rattled.

Then, almost from an unconscious place, I had the thought that I could go to the 24-hour grocery store down the street. Like that was going to solve something. It was a completely illogical thought. I didn't need groceries, and I had a full day ahead of me in the morning. Why would I do that? Then, I recognized it.

My old coping mechanism had arisen under a moment of stress and isolation. The urge to run. It was very similar to the live-wire feeling I had that night in my cottage in Northern California. An echo of an old reflex that brought the words, "I have to go". I was 20 when I actually followed through on that urge, packing up and leaving a home and region I loved.

On this night, though, I was 40 years old. I lived in a place I was deeply committed to; I was a mother, an educator, and an organization leader. I had my health and a network of long-time friends. Here, I want to share what I consider to be a small signal of triumph on the road to healing: I could look lovingly at the part of myself that had survived on those kinds of thoughts, and just hold it.

It was uncomfortable. The strongest shell of myself had to hold firm and breathe through the old pain. I had to get up and move my body to process the energy that was coursing through me. I danced and stretched in the dark of the big, open living room for most of an hour. There was an anguish in not getting to relieve the discomfort by running. I was reliving the pain of how school leaders had treated me, enduring new pain through current leaders, and welcoming strangers into my process. It added up to an understandable overwhelm. Yet, I had come this far... I could do this.

When I speak of the wound, the impacted place, I see it as a moment in the long arc of what unfolds afterward. If we survive, we adopt a **coping mechanism** - one to prevent future pain or one to make current pain more manageable. Sometimes both. Then, we get a respite while we live out the benefits, and eventually the costs, of that coping strategy.

Soon, though, because every living thing insists on ultimate health, we reach a **constriction** phase - where our coping mechanism starts to work against us. That which has kept us safe is now starting to destroy us. We've outgrown its effectiveness and need to shed it like a skin to keep living. I believe every transformation has death standing in wait, to give a nod of acknowledgment as we pass through the gate to rebirth. It is the one who takes the old skin, the too-small ideas or behaviors, as we expand into a next diameter of living. These are the trade-offs we make, the toll we pay, and the test of courage to stand naked and raw long enough to emerge new and exalted on the other side.

This part is tough, because it looks and feels like our lives are falling apart. Only, we have not failed. We are growing.

Next comes the **confrontation** - where we have to face the pain that evoked the coping mechanism, *and* the pain we may have caused by our clinging to it for temporary safety. This is the forged-in-the-fire part, where we grow a new layer of strength over all that had been before. I imagine those Russian nesting dolls, where the smaller doll is soon encircled by a seemingly identical, but larger and more robust next doll. The latest one holds all of them inside and is always the strongest of all yet.

Then, our **triumph** is not a one mountain-peak experience (much as we'd like it to be). It is small pivot points that lead to a new destination. It is moments of *choosing something other* than the coping mechanism and accepting whatever comes in its wake. These new choices start out as incredibly awkward or uncomfortable and soon become smooth and liberating.

Healing, or **transformation**, is when we reach renewal - we see differently than we did at the initial moment of impact - and can look back lovingly, appreciating ourselves for making the journey of the long arc to this point.

By about 1 am, I finally slept. In the morning, I submitted my Editorial with all the necessary corrections. I remembered who I was and how far I'd come, vividly enough to refocus and carry on.

OPINION

Burdensome choice is now Lawrence Academy's[9]

By **LOWELL SUN**

PUBLISHED: August 6, 2018 at 12:00 a.m. I UPDATED: July 11, 2019 at 12:00 a.m.

When I was 16, Lawrence Academy in Groton put me in a horrible position. Even more than failing to protect me from the child molester I had just confronted; even more than removing my sense of place and derailing my education, I was given the burdensome choice between allowing their decisions or honoring my conscience.

---

9 Vanessa Osage, The Lowell Sun, August 6, 2018, https://theamendsproject.com/press/

This is what honoring my conscience looks like: www.theamendsproject.com.

In 1994, Lawrence Academy decided to keep a documented child molester on campus after two students gave matching testimonies. In 2016, the school asked sex misconduct victims to step forward. Now, officials choose to "disagree" about any wrongdoing and are directing attention to a new investigation.

The choice to not settle with a former student, but instead hire private investigators to create an internal report to mitigate risk, is a clear message about the school's priorities...

It is time to resolve the persistent conflict of interest between Lawrence Academy to preserve a reputation — and of students and families for safety and protection. This is why I propose, and have created a model for, a Justice CORPS — the Committee to Oversee the Rights & Protections of Students.

My goal is to create a system that relieves my burden of addressing the wrongs done by an institution where adults within continually choose to do nothing. At 16, I made it my job to see that no further students would be harmed here in the same way. I need to hand over my burden now. I am ready for resolution.

Vanessa Osage, '96
www.theamendsproject.com

Diversion - Stay Focused

Of course, I flat-out refused to participate in that investigation. They were eagerly directing all attention away from their cover-up behaviors - past and present - and toward an employee long-gone. I also discovered that Elizabeth Sanghavi was a former associate at Holland & Knight, the law firm representing the school. As one former student wrote on social media, "I hope everyone can see this horse and pony show for what it is.".

They asked me repeatedly, over the course of many months, to give my story to their cause. Every time was a louder and more resounding NO.

When someone tries to divert attention away from the most pressing issue, we have to Stay Focused.

It is a test of attention and discipline. Of course, this is harder when the diversion is a personal attack or criticism. It is crucial to stand up for ourselves with a pointed fierceness, then keep energy concentrated on the goal. If we get caught up in defending ourselves, the diversion could succeed. So, efficiency is key. We must Stay Focused on our larger goal. The larger goal in this story is dismantling the persistent web of secrecy and silencing in these institutions.

The possibility of appearing on the Ellen Show fell away, and I did have some relief. But now, stepping off the legal path had birthed a practical solution. I had something tangible to promote beyond acknowledgment of the most valid point in need of repair. With my vision and my commitment to a humane approach to bringing it about, I could actively stay focused.

Warriors of Presence

"Being present allows us to access
the human resources of power,
presence and communication.
This is the way of the Warrior".

— Angeles Arrien, PhD

With Noah's help, I did what I could to prevent them from changing the subject. I continued to get emails from parents, with stories that devastated me anew, every time, even as the theme was not surprising to me. I dove into spending hours and hours on the phone with them, alumni, and parents of recent students, hearing their pain and distress.

Noah, who was still based in New England, was connecting with other former students, too. He fielded a similar kind of story one day. A classmate and friend of ours stopped by his home in Massachusetts to share his story of abuse by female employees at Lawrence Academy while he was a student there.

He was sexually abused by not one, but two employees on campus as a child. He told his father, who also worked at the school. Then, he found himself in an impossibly tight place, amidst unique and unexpected pressures.

One might think having a family member on campus would mean an assurance of justice for the child; only the opposite proved to be true.

Given the enduring culture of silencing on these campuses, right action (then or now) would actually disrupt his father's career. Imagine, doing right by children could be a threat to one's job security. This is the upside-down value system I refer to. The consequence at the time was these female employees were let go, without any warning to future employers.

With the situation left tragically unchecked, one of the abusive women continued to stalk my former classmate, well into his adulthood. My friend had always been understandably angry at the lack of accountability or consequence. Remember, **1 in 6 boys** are sexually abused during childhood. Then, when he heard my story in 2018, he had this new sense of guilt. Because he was male and a child of faculty, he still got to stay; he also didn't have to see the women who abused him on campus. Suddenly, to him, the contrast of my story made his experience seem less severe by comparison.

Of course, none of this is a burden that young people should have to shoulder under any circumstances. Disproportionate justice is its own secondary trauma, especially for people of character and conscience.

~ ~ ~

Noah and I talked regularly now. I have to give acknowledgment to the immense amount of time and care he gave to this cause. After Sybil, he became a most-enduring ally, especially that summer. Not all contact from former classmates was positive, though, and Noah became a solid source for clarity on that level, too. Soon, I sought his insights on what some negatively fixated on: the settlement amount.

I asked his opinion on the $500,000 figure since so many wanted to point to the financial compensation in a reflexive discrediting urge. The message from some was that my asking the institution to balance out my losses financially made me suspect. Never mind that the school's decision to keep a child molester on campus, remove me, and endanger others was most likely financially-based. Even with lowering my request to 25% of the attorney's demand, it became an easy focus for negative attention.

I asked Noah, "What do you think about the $500,000 amount?" He immediately brushed it aside with razor-sharp perspective. He said, "Look, if they give you a 500k settlement, that's still just... 1/52 of their endowment. These people put up buildings. That amount is nothing to them." He then made a highly valid point, "You have to keep in mind, their attorney is probably paid $500/hour from the school's funds to fight you off. So, the attorney is well-paid. It also means that the personal finances of each of the decision-makers are never touched by this situation." He spoke as someone who saw all sides with crystal clear focus.

He concluded, "By contrast, everything you put into reaching resolution comes at great, personal expense. You suffered as both a child who endured abuse and a visionary who was punished by adults. Don't think twice about that settlement amount". He was right.

Noah cared about justice, he cared about these schools, and he cared about each of us. He had actually contacted Lawrence Academy headmaster Dan Scheibe early on, just after the feature article came out. As a man who understood the law, Noah wanted to express his concerns over what he saw as "bad counsel" on behalf of the school's attorney. He had called, offering to help.

He spoke later to me about this, in exasperation over Dan Scheibe disregarding his offer. "They treat us no differently now than they would if we were still 15 years old.". I admired his strength to hold his love and care for all sides of this situation.

After the visit from our former classmate, Noah called to talk and unwind from the emotional upheaval. He joked, "Welcome to Vanessa's world.". He meant that now he had a taste of what I was living each day, with more and more people contacting me to share their anguish over how Lawrence Academy leaders were mistreating families.

~ ~ ~

I had to keep this on track. I also saw that by school leaders dodging responsibility for mishandling, former students were carrying a disproportionate share of the weight. While I was always happy to be present for those who needed it, I was increasingly aware of carrying the burden while they hid. This was not right. I started dreaming up a kind of press conference, where I could ask current leaders to show up and hold the responsibility as well. They needed to address these underlying issues that were so impacting students, alumni, parents, and more. I was responding. It was time for them to be present and face the wave of devastation that had surfaced as a result of their poor handling.

I'd coordinated nearly a dozen community events in my hometown of Bellingham, Washington, while Executive Director of Rooted Emerging. I knew how to weave resources together to create a meaningful moment for people. So, I got started on coordinating this event in the Boston area. I posted a Job Description on the Boston Facilitator's Roundtable, for a professional facilitator to oversee the event. I got a call from Abby Yanow, President of the organization. She was interested in the issue and willing to help.

She had a number of valid concerns about the length of time, the level of emotion in the attendees, and the goals for the time. Her expertise was priceless. We came up with an agenda that could fit an initial gathering, and she kept in touch as I continued to confirm details. Holding events at public libraries required charitable organization status - which I was yet to attain at that point. So, I found a venue called "The Green Room" in Cambridge, Massachusetts, and booked a time slot for the evening of August 16, 2018. The coordinator looked at my website, saw what I was doing, and became an active supporter. I needed the help, too, since I was doing all of this from the far other side of the country.

~ ~ ~

I was in touch with reporters and newscasters from all around Boston. People were interested. People were pissed. Of course, they wanted to hear what school leaders had to say about this. All kinds of people needed that.

On August 9, 2018, I invited Dan Scheibe and Bruce MacNeil:

Greetings Dan and Bruce,

I am writing to formally invite you both to a press conference on Wednesday August 15, 2018 to publicly address my concerns - along with those of many others - for resolution in the Amends Project.

Then, I followed up the day before the event.

Wed, Aug 15, 2018, 7:35 AM

to Dan, Bruce

On behalf of nearly a dozen outraged, concerned alumni and former staff, and in collaboration with multiple regional news outlets, you are formally called upon to attend a Public Response event:

Thursday August 16, 2018
6-7 pm
Prospect Hill
Somerville, Massachusetts

This invitation is intended solely for Lawrence Academy Headmaster Dan Scheibe, Trustee Bruce MacNeil and former Headmaster Steve Hahn. While you have the right to legal counsel on your own time, no attorney may be present at the event.

...Secondarily, I need a commitment to re-engage in a series of change-making talks for four consecutive weeks in October 2018. This allows a full six weeks for tempers to calm and positive action steps to become clearer.

Truly,

Vanessa Osage

When I got no response on August 15, I called Lawrence Academy to speak to Dan. The secretary told me, "He's in and out of the office today.". I said it was important that he get back to me as soon as possible. She said she would give him the message when she saw him.

I called again hours later, and the secretary told me he was in a meeting. I said, "You might want to interrupt that meeting." Then, after a long hold, she actually got back on the line and said to me, "Um, I mean, he is on vacation.". I smirked in sarcasm, "On vacation from me, or actually on vacation?". Her voice sped up in nervousness, "On vacation." I hung up.

Rick was standing by. I called and told him what I heard. He did some work in the newsroom and said, "We have a story.".

NEWS LATEST HEADLINES

Woman who says she was molested at Lawrence Academy in the '90s holding public response event[10]

By **RICK SOBEY**
PUBLISHED: August 15, 2018 at 12:00 a.m. I UPDATED: July 11, 2019 at 12:00 a.m.

SOMERVILLE — The Lawrence Academy alumna who says she was sexually molested by a school worker in the 1990s has organized a "public response event" for Thursday.

---

[10] Rick Sobey, The Lowell Sun, August 15, 2018, https://theamendsproject.com/press/

At the event in Somerville, Vanessa (Fadjo) Osage will call on school leaders to address concerns of "covering up child sexual abuse at the institution," she said Wednesday.

...School officials will not attend, according to a statement from Lawrence Academy on Wednesday.

"From the message calling on representatives of the school to attend the event, it is our understanding that its purpose is to pressure the School to change its response to and valuation of the former student's claims," reads the school's statement. "As we have said publicly, we have carefully and respectfully considered each request from this alumna and responded in ways that we believe are reasonable and appropriate."...

"Unfortunately, communications with this alumna have become increasingly less constructive and the proposals she has generated have become less reasonable," reads the statement. "We do not feel the circumstances around the proposed event on August 16th demonstrate good faith that would lead to a productive result."

... [the article mentions the "disagreement" as well as the investigation by Sanghavi Group]

Some of Osage's former classmates have recently reached out to the school, expressing outrage about how they've handled the situation.

Marguerite Bryant, for instance, wrote to the school: "Vanessa would have had a very different life if she hadn't experienced this trauma at the hands of those meant to protect and educate her."

Leah Jarkko, from the Class of 1997, wrote to school leaders: "Earn the trust of those children and families, of your staff by acknowledging wrongdoing and pledging to support to making positive change and rectifying mishandling of past administrations."

The Thursday event open to the public is planned for 6 p.m. at the Green Room studio, 62 Bow St., Somerville.

Discrediting & Defamation - Be Who You Are

The remedy for Discrediting or Defamation seems simple, yet it is profound in the long term: Be Who You Are.

Actions will always speak loudest. We can trust in the intelligence of people to see the reality of a situation over time. Our choices reveal us more than anything. Lawrence Academy leaders made a few clear and revealing choices. Noah and I kept in touch as the evening unfolded in a frenzy... They didn't show.

When he saw the article from August 15, Noah called (very late for him) to console and give perspective. He said, "Rick Sobey's got a series. It's part of their approach in journalism to make each party the bad guy at some point.". Noah also was aghast at the overstep by Bruce MacNeil. "This is dangerously close to defamation.", he commented. We added it to a tally of legal offenses they were accumulating. It was a new low.

A friend on the west coast read the article and said, "If I didn't know you, and read this, I would think you were crazy.". That's the point of defamation, after all. Noah said, "You have endured institutional abuse, first privately, and now publicly". He also insisted on reminding me that something had begun here, and I was up to the challenge of seeing it through.

His calm, steady wisdom definitely kept me going at that point, exhausted as I was.

The next day, I contacted Bruce MacNeil. *Being Who You Are* is strengthened by naming our motivations, values, and goals - and following these with action. We can confront the behavior for what it is, and then illustrate the context of the situation. We don't stoop to lower levels. We name it without becoming it. That means keeping enough ethical distance from the behavior to still be ourselves. Sometimes, we are the musician and the sudden caller of the missteps. Then we pick up our instrument and play our song again. This is one of the many gifts of friendship: collaboration to help us remember our truest rhythm and refrain.

Courage / Leadership

Aug 16, 2018, 4:11 PM

Bruce,

I would like to speak with you over the phone.

If you have the courage, I invite you to call me at 3 pm EST tomorrow, Friday August 17.

Vanessa

Aug 17, 2018, 7:58 AM

Vanessa,

I am not available for a call. As I wrote in my email of August 1, please direct any further communication to Dan and Libby.

Regards,

Bruce MacNeil

Fri, Aug 17, 2018, 9:23 AM

to Dan, Bruce

Bruce,

You have never met or even spoken to me. Yet you feel entitled to criticize my character publicly. Now, you deny my request for a phone conversation…

Well, true to form, every bully is a coward (at least temporarily) at heart.

You seem to forgot you are leaders of an organization that cares for kids.

Parents see how you are handling me - a student harmed under your care - and they hold their babies a little closer to their chest.

Alumni have started cautioning families with young teens against considering Lawrence Academy. They are unnerved by how you have responded to me since coming forward, again.

As for the continued abuse of language, let's look at your "unreasonable" comment.

I am, in fact, able to share my reasoning around the demands (reason-able). They are quite simple.

My reason for adding an additional resolution point was that I discovered a young man very close to current administration had been allowed (quite recently) to go on to sexually assault more young women, with zero safety check for anyone involved.

The reason I added this point is that people are trusting ME with their stories (curious, how is cooperation from alumni going in your investigation?). I have been holding numerous horrible stories of young people abused and then silenced at Lawrence Academy.

The reason I added this additional point is because I feel a moral obligation to take action to see that no further harm is suffered by young people on their path to a successful adult life...

You?

Remember also, this tactic of intimidating and mistreating me in hopes of getting me/my message to go away has not worked for you yet. Not in 1994, not in 2001, not now in 2018.

"Let's do the right thing here" and
"Go away. We're fine."

is becoming an awfully old and worn-out conversation.

My invitation to a new kind of conversation (unscripted by attorneys, out from behind closed doors) remains open to you.

You know my goals:

1. bring the truth to light
2. hold school leaders to account
3. enact lasting, positive change

Do let me know if you find good reason to join me in this effort.

Vanessa Osage, '96

p.s. yes, I will cc Dan here, and continue the conversation with him.

The Double-Talk Shuffle

"It doesn't matter how many times
you get knocked down.
All that matters is you get up
one more time than you were knocked down."

— Roy T. Bennett

I coordinated one more event at The Green Room in Somerville, Massachusetts. Even with the weird previous outcome, a number of new people had been drawn into the effort and craved a new forum for connecting. I collaborated closely with Abby Yanow, who gave crucial structure to guiding for the long view of the process.

Our Kids' Needs First

The Power of Honest Conversations Series

Hosted by The Amends Project

All families deserve the assurance of knowing that,
if anything happened to their child at school,
the needs and wellbeing of the child would absolutely come first.

Join us for a follow-up conversation, generated by interest
in the Public Response Event of August 16.
Welcoming concerned parents to an open forum
with Lawrence Academy alumni and associates to discuss the issues.
Come, learn about The Justice CORPS proposal and more.
Be a part of enacting lasting, positive change
for the protection of all students.

Friday August 31, 2018
5:30-7:30 pm
The Green Room
Somerville, MA

~ ~ ~

Just before my announcing this follow-up event, The New York Times published an article:

"Catholic Priests Abused 1,000 Children in Pennsylvania, Report Says"[11]

By Laurie Goodstein and Sharon Otterman

Bishops and other leaders of the Roman Catholic Church in Pennsylvania covered up child sexual abuse by more than 300 priests over a period of 70 years, persuading victims not to report the abuse and law enforcement not to investigate it, according to **a searing report issued by a grand jury** on Tuesday.

---

[11] Laurie Goodstein & Sharon Otternam, The New York Times, August 14, 2018, https://www.nytimes.com/2018/08/14/us/catholic-church-sex-abuse-pennsylvania.html

...The sexual abuse scandal has shaken the Catholic Church for more than 15 years, ever since explosive allegations emerged out of Boston in 2002. But even after paying billions of dollars in settlements and adding new prevention programs, the church has been dogged by a scandal that is now reaching its highest ranks.

... But several bishops, including Bishop David A. Zubik of Pittsburgh, rejected the idea the church had concealed abuse.

"There was no cover-up going on," Bishop Zubik said in a news conference on Tuesday. "I think that it's important to be able to state that. We have over the course of the last 30 years, for sure, been transparent about everything that has in fact been transpiring."

Church officials followed a "playbook for concealing the truth," the grand jury said, minimizing the abuse by using words like "inappropriate contact" instead of "rape"; assigning priests untrained in sexual abuse cases to investigate their colleagues; and not informing the community of the real reasons behind removing an accused priest.

..."I had gone to two bishops with allegations over five years, and they ignored and downplayed my allegations," said the Rev. James Faluszczak, an Erie priest on extended leave who was abused as a child and who testified before the grand jury. "It's that very management of secrets that has given cover to predators."

For others, it was too little, too late. Frances Samber, whose brother Michael was abused by a priest in Pittsburgh and committed suicide in 2010, said, "It's good that the public sees this, but where is the justice? What do you do about it? Why aren't these people in prison?"

. . . "They wanted to cover up the cover-up," said Mr. Shapiro, the attorney general.

~ ~ ~

Dan Scheibe had made an unverified claim to The Lowell Sun in May, "Scheibe said the school did not, and would never, withhold financial aid as a retaliatory measure. He added the school cannot comment on any one case because financial support is confidential."

Words were thrown over their shoulders, like a maze of tangles in the wake of one trying to outrun the truth - and avoid the necessity of true healing.

~ ~ ~

Then, a beautiful irony played out at summer's end. Lawrence Academy made a post on their social media, right on the heels of asking people to participate in their investigation. I didn't see either one - being intentionally off their mailing list and not on social media. What I saw, though, was a new tsunami of activity in response to the obvious hypocrisy.

It seemed, Lawrence Academy officials were quick to believe their word had surpassed all public attention on The Amends Project; that they had effectively gotten rid of me with the last low blow of defamation to the press. You might say, a certain arrogance over their ability to sway public opinion came up once again - the old Achillea's Heel. By September, they started tripping over themselves with the public outrage over the double message.

One alumna posted on Facebook (and a friend emailed me a screenshot):

"To post this the same week as they sent that letter is tone deaf as hell. It's shameful what happened while we were there. It's shameful how they handled it. It's just plain ridiculous that they just can't seem to get it right now. Until they put our classmate first, I strongly suggest we withhold all forms of alumni giving. It's really more than unfortunate that as significant a role that Lawrence Academy played in shaping who I've become- that now I won't even consider sending my son there!!!"

People were not fooled.

The Franciscan Monk, Father Richard Rohr, speaks to what he has witnessed as a "father hunger" at the root of so many social ills affecting our culture. He says, "When positive masculine energy is not modeled from father to son, it creates a vacuum in the souls of men, and into that vacuum, demons pour. Among other things, they seem to lose the ability to know how to read situations and people clearly."

Would people still invest great financial resources in a tuition where school leaders defame a former student? How would you read that situation? It's not the oil industry we're looking at, not stock trading, or gold prospecting - it's a school. Lawrence Academy, like all private, independent high schools, is a business. It depends on the choice of families to buy into their ($52,000 - $65,000/year) services.

It operates on the premise that they provide an exceptionally good experience for kids and families. Business is relationships. Are we acting as wise consumers when we ignore this problem, or get caught up in the reminder of how low their acceptance rate is? If more people are applying than the school accepts as students, does that fact guarantee quality alone?

The Power of Honest Conversations continued; only it became loud and amplified over social media. I didn't have to coordinate long-distance events, after all. Thanks to an old friend, conversations flew over these channels with such force that Lawrence Academy was reeling from the constant ripples in their pond. This old friend was good enough to keep me informed with continuous updates and screenshots.

As the school year began, former classmates started commenting on Lawrence Academy's social media posts. Pictures of new freshmen in get-to-know-you games inspired, "Trust falls indeed". Every post included a link to The Amends Project website. A classmate started a petition for people to pledge to not give money to the school until they made my situation right. Of course, what people wanted most of all - to my understanding - was the necessary relief of a once-trusted institution demonstrating worthiness of that trust.

A new email from another former student gave me insight into sentiment around school communications, and the cover-up culture.

Hi Vanessa,

I'm not sure if you'll remember me…

When I got the email from LA a few weeks ago regarding your story, it didn't sit right with me. Something just seemed off. My sister, who graduated two years before me, felt the same way. When I read about your story today I instantly knew why. They were trying to cover their butt and that came through in the email.

As someone who was also abused as a child, I am SO proud of you. Knowing exactly what you'd be facing by coming forward, and doing it anyway, is an incredibly brave thing to do. I just wanted to let you know that you are making a difference for so many young (and older!) people. Thank you for being an honest, brave, and compassionate person.

I thanked her, and she wrote again, offering to share her own experience.

Your story is really stirring up some old feelings that I have from my time there. So, I'll share my own awful experience with the LA administration.

Near the end of junior year I told a female administrator, who was also my Advisor, that I was suicidal. While I sobbed on the couch in her office, she collected a bunch of brochures from other schools and asked me which one I wanted to transfer to. A few days later, Steve Hahn called my mother and told her I wasn't invited back for senior year. My grades were fine and I hadn't gotten into any trouble so we were confused. I don't recall what bullshit excuse Hahn gave my mom, but she hit the ROOF. When I returned for senior year, the teachers and staff basically ignored me.

That was the darkest time of my life. I reached out for help to not only be rejected, but to also be actively disposed of.

Each one of these stories re-energized me. First, I felt the agony and then renewed energy for action. This was why I was persisting on this path. Noah had suggested we create a Facebook page for The Amends Project. I said, If someone was willing to coordinate and set it up, I would learn how to work within it. Late that summer, a social media presence arrived, and former students joined as "friends". I learned to watch posts on the "wall" and, most especially, to participate in private conversations out of view inside Messaging.

A few students were actively pursued by the Sanghavi Group to participate in the school's investigation. It had intensified when they commented on The Amends Project Facebook page. Some started to feel negatively preyed upon. So, the conversation went underground.

It was wild, potent, and sometimes unruly exchange. Big feelings surfaced, sometimes flaring into rage and lashings-out. Then, others were able to respond skillfully, addressing the feelings beneath the behavior, and folding them back into what I would call love. There was tenderness, too, while everyone dealt with grieving their trust and facing a new truth. It was an honest, pseudo-human-connection theatre like I had never witnessed.

I felt a responsibility to keep the focus on long-range goals and intentions: Where we are going, and how we will get there. My experience as the leader of a nonprofit became relevant here.

I laid these out and watched people reference them in tough moments.

Goals of The Amends Project:

1. Bring the truth to light.

2. Hold leaders accountable.
3. Enact lasting, positive change.

Core Tenets of The Amends Project:

1. No further exploitation will be allowed on the way toward resolution.
2. Success by means of fear/control is no success at all.
3. Situations will be influenced only by the sheer power of honesty, a fierce insistence on accountability, and the encouragement toward true growth and positive change.
4. The Project will only conclude when leaders admit to the cover up, and new policies are firmly in place to protect the rights and wellbeing of students for perpetuity.
5. This is for everyone.

Destruction & Rebirth

"The reasonable wo/man adapts
her/himself to the world:
the unreasonable one persists in trying
to adapt the world to her/himself.
Therefore all progress depends
on the unreasonable wo/man."

— George Bernard Shaw

"In chaos, there is fertility."

— Anais Nin

I had to move residences again, and the energy of keeping this movement for transparency and accountability afloat was taking its toll in my life. I had conviction. I had resourcefulness. I had energy and support and, most importantly, I had a vision. I did not have housing stability or steady income. I'd been self-employed for over a decade. So, with no settlement from the school, I had a new challenge upon me.

How was I going to balance the influx of contact from alumni and parents, advance The Justice CORPS, and still support myself?

Giving the people who reached out my time was a choice I was making. The idea of charging for my coaching and consulting on this issue was beyond conceivable. I felt such a heart-level impulse to be present for them. They had woken up from the "big lie" and I'd known that pain from various angles, through so many stages of my life. Loving response to our need to understand and be understood is such a balm for our humanity. Especially when you've been pushed into a unique kind of isolation, I knew, it was crucial for health.

~ ~ ~

Yet, for balance, I had to find the discipline to shift my focus: from tending the emotional upheaval this brings for people - to employing my Executive Director skill set and making real progress on The Justice CORPS. It was hard to do. I'd just traveled down to Marysville, WA - midway between Bellingham and Seattle - to meet an old classmate who lived in the city now. He was fired-up and very focused, with a great east-coast sensibility that brought an anchor to my vision of creating lasting change.

The issue was deeply personal for him, since his mother had sat on the Board of Trustees, and he'd grown up with these players in close contact during his childhood. The closer they are to you, the more devastation when you learn this truth. He'd suggested we alumni gather on the Lawrence Academy campus for Open House, which was coming up in less than two months. He talked about ways to focus energy and delegate tasks to people. He was clear, organized, straightforward, and also kind. I felt blessed to have an in-person, west-coast ally.

He'd also recognized that I was nearing burn out. I was sweating through some fever when I met him, and as I said, I'd recently moved. It took a caring old connection to say, "Hey, you need to take a break.". He assured me that he and a few others could carry it while I rested. I would need my strength. So, I set up the Action Plan, checked in with the most vocal participants, and pulled myself away from the action to sleep and reorient to my life.

When that kind of wave rises up under your feet, touching ground again can take time and real determination.

It's important to say - this was a concentrated effort *for* transparency, accountability, and change. It was not against one school, or even a few individuals. Defense tactics were slamming up against reveal-the-truth efforts and tensions played out. Depending on where people were in their process, some got amplified in the anger stage. This was understandable, especially when the realization came after years of buried memories, stored like trauma, with no outlet for release for decades. We were all moving through grief stages, since we'd lost both an illusion and faith in a core segment of society.

People wanted different things. The intentions kept the collective focused. Yet, we have to honor the timing of the process that is so unique to each person. Along those lines, there were moments when conflicting desires were expressed. Yes, I wanted restitution and lasting, positive change - root level change in response. Some people, in part-truth, part-joke, said they just wanted arson.

I thought to the very early history of the school, *"An errant firecracker set fire to the Groton, Massachusetts School Building in 1868". Two years later, women were denied entry - contradicting the publicly stated intention to provide for "the education of both sexes" . They were prevented from attending for almost 100 years. Then, another major fire struck in 1956, during the boys-only years. Young women were granted entry again by 1971 . . .*

It does make you wonder about patterns of destruction and rebirth.

~ ~ ~

The cultural backdrop on this planning phase in The Amends Project was the Kavanaugh nomination and hearing. I'd never followed a news story so closely. Justice Brett Kavanaugh had been nominated to the Supreme Court by Donald Trump in July 2018. Then, a psychology professor in California, Dr. Christine Blassey-Ford, felt a moral obligation to speak on what she knew of Kavanaugh, personally.

At age 15, she alleged, Brett Kavanaugh had tried to rape her at a party, physically assaulting her and covering her face to the point that she feared she might not survive. The issue of abortion rights and the pro-life debate weighed heavily on this nomination - a women's physical sovereignty issue at its heart. Supreme Court appointments are lifelong positions, so the stakes were high.

Dr. Blassey-Ford spoke out. The world watched.

This tension surfaced all of the unconscious biases and beliefs we, as Americans, had about the weight of sexual assault, and how that behavior colors professional character. We had let an alleged rapist make it to the highest office in the land, after all. It was time to start working our way back down the hierarchy ladder and restructure a new value system onto the whole process.

In September, I was fully in transition for housing and, at a strange, new low in meeting my basic needs. Another alumna started a petition to help me continue in this effort, and the donations paid my rent and grocery bills more than once. I recall sitting with my car full of houseplants, waiting for the temporary rental in the Lettered Streets neighborhood to be ready for my entry. I drove down to the Marina, parked by a friend's van, which held my other things, and listened to NPR coverage while my life was on hold.

Just hearing those tensions in the voices of commentators brought me a funny sense of relief. It was about damn time we were talking about this. Talking calmly and honestly about sexuality was a big part of my professional life at that point. I'd been teaching Comprehensive Sexuality Education to ages 6 & up for many years, in addition to coaching and consulting. I knew the great relief and appreciation people would feel with the freedom to share something so personal and meaningful. It was one of the sweetest rewards of my work.

So, my primary reaction to these broadcasts was, *'Hallelujah, welcome to the conversation!'*. We, as Americans, got to watch how internal defenses played out in a public forum. It was *Fascinating*. Of course, men had always found ways to justify this behavior - actions that were either encouraged or shunned, depending on the audience. It's all enough to confuse a boy, about what it means to be a real man.

Now, people in America (and beyond) got to take a plain look at the emotional reactions to a woman asserting her rights for bodily autonomy, safety, and the dignity of choice. The country's president actually mocked her before an audience. Yet, now we also had to face that those physical boundaries had been hers all along. So glad we could finally clear that up. How was it, that a man who others thought so highly of could also enact violence against a young woman, in front of a male friend... and still conclude himself, a 'good man'? We all needed to start sorting this out NOW.

Blassey-Ford and Kavanaugh did. They helped us start the process. Every conversation their hearing inspired was worthwhile because it brought these questions into awareness. Of course, I wanted an outcome of justice and accountability, too. Let's be clear - I did not believe the man worthy of the position, given the (multiple) allegations or the inhuman response to a fellow human being. I could stand behind no man who would pretend in such a sphere, when the whole world would count on his integrity as a potential judge. He did not allow his humanity to show up to the conversation once. Sensitivity for his own plight, yes. But decency toward a woman who risked naming a horrible act as horrible? The man's response was only denial and disregard. That was not Supreme Court Judge-character, in my assessment.

Again, from Richard Rohr, "I think the truly human is always experienced in vulnerability, in mutuality, in reciprocity. When human beings try to deny their own vulnerability, even from themselves, when they cannot admit weakness, neediness, hurt, pain, suffering, sadness, they become very unhuman and not very attractive. They don't change you; they don't invite you."

Because of my commitment to truth-telling, I felt moved by the significance of the moment. I was hopeful. The conversation gave new messages to young boys trying to decipher that tricky "real man" question. It gave new information to young women who might have no context on what "normal" or "healthy" handling was in private, sexual moments. Brett Kavanaugh was brought to account, but not yet held to account. That's where we were. As a culture, we were not yet strong enough to lift it to where it all belonged.

But, it was a Beginning.

Oversight - This is for Everyone

"Our capacity to destroy one another
is matched by our capacity to heal one another...
We can change social conditions to
create environments in which children and adults
can feel safe and where they can thrive."

— Bessel van der Kolk, MD

It just didn't have to be this way. It didn't have to be silence and secrecy and hiding. Because, as Trevor Noah says, society is a contract we make with each other, we can simply write up a new contract. Every social construct can be pieced apart and remade in a new image of health

By October, 2018, I was settled into my new, cozy cottage and focusing primarily on developing The Justice CORPS model. I was making new professional connections with experts and advocates around the country to enhance this vision. Their insights and feedback helped me adjust the model toward greater and greater effectiveness. Soon, I welcomed my first Professional Advisor, Justine Finn of Relation-Shift, at the Harvard Innovation Lab. The mission for her project was "End Sexual Violence. Promote Healthy Relationships. Create Safer Schools".

I love the magic that happens when you hop into the positively creative, interconnected system that courses beneath our world. When people work together with a common spirit and vision, all movement becomes enhanced by the synergy. Justine understood the path to reform better than anyone I'd met yet. It is always a gift to connect with someone who speaks your language and walks a similar path.

A new development arose in the ongoing expose of New England boarding schools, which validated my calls for oversight in response to abuse. Friends and supporters in The Amends Project would send me all kinds of news . . .

Overseer to work with St. Paul's after criminal investigation[12]

By Laura Crimaldi GLOBE STAFF | SEPTEMBER 13, 2018, 2:21 p.m.

A 14-month investigation into St. Paul's School found enough evidence to charge the school with endangering the welfare of children, the New Hampshire attorney general's office announced Thursday.

. . . Attorney General Gordon J. MacDonald revealed the findings during an afternoon news conference at his office in Concord.

"We could have charged the school," MacDonald said.
Instead, MacDonald said, he has signed an agreement with St. Paul's School to appoint an overseer to work at the school for five years.

"Rather we pursued a course of comprehensive reform," MacDonald said. Criminal charges would, at most, have resulted in misdemeanor convictions and fines, he said.

---

12 Laura Crimaldi, The Boston Globe, September 13, 2018, https://www.bostonglobe.com/metro/2018/09/13/unprecedented-agreement-resolve-criminal-investigation-into-paul-school/BK4kUhKS3nPWBsO1YxwE8N/story.html

The overseer will report to the New Hampshire Department of Justice and will enforce the agreement between St. Paul's School and the attorney general. Public reports will be required on a biannual basis.

The agreement requires St. Paul's School to report alleged abuse of students to the overseer and the New Hampshire Department of Justice before launching an internal investigation, MacDonald said.

This was thrilling because my concept of oversight in The Justice CORPS had made its way into consciousness as a higher response to mishandling of abuse on high school campuses. It also challenged the validity of internal investigations, whether called "independent" by schools or not. I reached out to Gordon MacDonald (who had already been on my list of potential allies) to ask if he was willing to endorse The Justice CORPS. I did not get a response, but his decision with St. Paul's gave me encouragement to keep going, trusting in the necessity of an oversight model.

~ ~ ~

I understood that my personal conflict with decision-makers at Lawrence Academy would keep some potential allies at a distance. Taking a stand on an issue in a broad sense can feel safer than taking a stand in the tension between two parties. Larger principles show up in the sharpest relief in those personal conflicts - yet, somehow, people have been hesitant to "take sides". What do we stand for, or who do we stand for... and how might we stand on more solid ground?

This had also played out in the Blassey-Ford/Kavanaugh encounter.

I continued to remain resolute on combining restitution with reform, for a number of reasons. I came to each of these through a lot of introspection, contemplation, and soul-searching. This, from a post I made later that year, with my reasons:

Core Tenet # 5 of The Amends Project is **"This is for everyone"**. *How so?*

Simply put, I will take no conclusion that benefits me and offers no lasting change to support others. Likewise, I will accept no outcome that benefits everyone else and excludes myself.

This is for everyone.

Of course, The Justice CORPS is designed to benefit more and more families in schools, and eventually churches – then, someday – other structures of power.

If, for some, the right and best answer is to confidentially accept a tuition waiver, or to go to court and receive confidential settlement – I give my full acceptance.

Everyone's path is unique, and I expect no one to mimic my path if it goes against what they know is right for them. I also believe that everyone is called to make a stand – in some way – in some aspect of their lives, at some point, to become fully whole and human. It may be confronting an abusive parent, or standing up for themselves to an employer, or refusing to participate in a system that destroys something they hold valuable. Each meets their own.

This just happens to be mine.

As a brilliant colleague pointed out, when this school can settle with me in the context of honesty, respect and fairness – it sets a precedent for other people who may ever encounter an abuse of power of any kind. It will be an offering to the world that says, "It can be done."

This is for Everyone. This means what benefits others must also benefit the one giving the gift.

Yes, generosity is a remarkable virtue where the joy and benefit truly can lie in the giving alone. It creates more and sustains the heart and soul. "It is in giving that we receive', it is said. Of course, there are *many* places in life that call for a pure and altruistic giving. Places of trust, established reciprocity and love. Wisdom reminds us that anywhere an imbalance of power and resources is currently causing harm, generosity must be tempered.

There is a necessary wisdom in giving well.

As Lynn Twist beautifully says, "If you're in touch with the pain and suffering in this world, and you're really willing to open your heart to that – you will do something about it. You will do what's yours to do. And, in order to do what's your to do and to do it well, you need to take care of yourself, too."

I have slowly learned over decades that I have to include myself in my generosity toward the world. If I give to others at the expense of myself, there has truly been a less-than-ideal exchange. If you're real with yourself, you know where you currently fall on this continuum… Also, and this is an indicator of healing on many levels, *reclaiming inclusion in the good of the world is an antidote to being excluded for speaking up for what is right.*

When two people are negotiating for fair conclusion, or seeking to find the middle ground, both positions have equal value in stating their needs. **I am showing up to this table in full possession of my equal value.**

What's happening in The Amends Project is a rebalancing of order and power. There are larger principles at play.

Fiduciary Responsibility, as one alumna put it.

Accountability, as many have echoed.

Justice, as so many relate to this.

So, I am also unwilling to give an inconsistent message. If I make my efforts solely about other people and other schools without insisting on honest, positive resolution in my situation – I have added a coin to the piggy bank of complacency. I am not making that investment.

Most importantly, I proceed with a balance of This is for Everyone, because, as a mentor, teacher, coach and guide to young and old, I always remember that my very life is a teaching tool. To be effective in my life's work, I have to live in alignment with my values, knowing that my actions speak far louder than my words. I teach by how I live. In this, I would not ever say to a young person embarking on a journey for social justice, "Spend decades of your life working to right wrongs and protect those around you, but deny your own needs and experience." No.

I would only ever say to a young person in my care, "Yes, spend as long as it takes to see that you get the results you know in your heart are necessary to make this world a better, safer place. And, you absolutely remember this – defend your own rights, needs and wellbeing along the way."

On the Culture of a Place

"Frightened men behave
as if the truth were not true."

— Bayard Rustin

With my new focus of attention, I began to feel more at home in my "work" again. I knew how to collaborate for a larger vision - how to draw on the skills of many, and weave them into something greater than any one of us. It was what sustained me in creating my first nonprofit from 2009-2019, and my soul smiled at knowing this work was a new experience of home for me.

I continued to get messages from people I didn't know, those who were compelled to reach me and corroborate the issue. One story deserves special attention here: the most recent cover-up from Lawrence Academy yet. I've been given permission to share this family's story from 2017.

The email from the mother read:

October 13, 2018

We are interested in contacting Vanessa Osage or her attorneys about her legal claims with LA. We have a son who was enrolled at Lawrence Academy 16/17 and feel our insight may be helpful. Unrelated, my sisters and I both attended Nobles 1987- -1990, And I grew up in Concord Ma.

I emailed to set a time to talk, and she told me her family's ordeal...

Her son left his home in the midwest, at age 14, to attend Lawrence Academy for his freshman year in 2016. Like her email said, this mother had attended Nobles (Noble & Greenough, a sectarian boarding school for grades 7 - 12 in Dedham, Massachusetts). The family made the choice to give him this experience because the boy's father was having health issues, and the parents were so distracted by medical appointments and logistics; they wanted to spare him the stress. They believed starting at Lawrence Academy would give him an enriching, carefree experience.

But, a few months into the year, her son was in a class where a teacher had assigned reading with a graphic description of a character's surgery as a result of breast cancer. The boy's grandmother had recently died of breast cancer, so he became very emotional at reading this. He got up suddenly and walked to the restroom down the hall. He didn't want to cry in front of his new classmates. The teacher then (apparently ego-affronted that he'd left without asking), allegedly stormed into the bathroom after him - grabbed him by the back of his collar and physically dragged him back to class.

The boy told his mother, who was naturally upset.

The mother then contacted administration to make a complaint. What she found was not a "firm pledge to a resolve of care". Dan Scheibe and other school officials minimized her concerns and said glibly; they would "look into it". They eventually came back with a story of the teacher's defense, claiming that he'd "tripped" while in the boys' bathroom. An issue of excessive gravity, he'd suggested.

Of course, the mother did not accept this excuse or fabrication. She also rejected the lack of care in response by administrators. This was her 14 year-old son, away from home for the first time. So she flew out to Groton, Massachusetts - all the way from the midwest - to talk with them in person.

She told me they were still evasive and dismissing. She said she sat in that office with Dan Scheibe, Libby Margraf, and a few others, and said very clearly that she expected corrective action. She described the blank stares, all stunned into a frightened silence and unwilling to act.

Scheibe offered her a tuition refund if she simply withdrew her son from school. What is the difference between this response and the stories of Steve Hahn in the 1990s? This is where the "one year of tuition" as compensation comes back around in the larger story. Paul Lannon offered me (as an adult in 2018) the equivalent of one year's tuition - not adjusted for inflation - from the 1990s: $25,000. At this point, with Dan Scheibe as headmaster in 2017, we're talking about $65,000 as payment in advance of legal action. A refund with your forced-exit is not my idea of "progress". Of course, this mother was already invested financially and practically in her son's education. She shouldn't have to face that kind of decision. She was irate.

"No, I am not going to just take him out of school! It's your responsibility to address this assault with the teacher who did it and make sure my son is safe on campus!" she told them. This was hardly a year before Dan Scheibe made the public statement in May 2018, "However, in the present day of Lawrence Academy, we have consistently taken action to ensure our campus is a safe environment in which students can thrive with a sense of protection and security."

Then, in a spirit I both recognize and appreciate, this mother just kept talking about it. She'd show up at Trustee meetings and voice her concerns, or contact other parents on the Parents Association. She would reach out to people on campus directly. She became a constant reminder of that discrepancy between word and action. She spoke up and kept speaking up for her family's right to receive decent treatment, following abuse by an adult employee on campus.

When I talked about meeting Dan Scheibe in person earlier that year, after they'd cancelled our agreed-upon Restorative Justice Circle in February, she asked with a laugh, "Did he look nervous?" He had, indeed, I told her. She continued, "I'd been in his office, on the phone, and complaining to anyone who would listen about all of this.". I felt I'd met a predecessor and an ally, just priming the pump for me without my even realizing. She might have been insistently in conversation Dan Scheibe right about the time Mitchell Garabedian sent that demand letter for $2 million. I felt my own sense of gratitude.

This mother told me on the phone, "My experience at these schools was largely positive when I was a kid, and if someone had told me one of these stories at the time, I don't think I would have believed them...". She admitted, "I might have thought they were crazy or making it up." Then, she said, with what I've come to recognize as a unique mix of disappointment and anger, "But now, I know.".

She had become an ardent spokesperson about the injustice of their inadequate response, no matter the social costs for speaking. I said something to her about a 'culture of fear,' and she gave an emphatic, "Yes! That's exactly what it is.". This mother was making all this noise about unethical handling of abuse on campus while Mitchell Garabedian and I were preparing to move forward with a lawsuit. When she and I spoke, she told me her family was also considering legal action against the school.

Like all the others, she expressed gratitude for my speaking out about the ways officials at Lawrence Academy of Groton, Massachusetts, sought to silence families and conceal the facts about abuse on campus.

Her son did finish out his freshman year, largely on the principle that he should not have to leave because of one abusive staff person. It was a principle I had lived out in my life, as my own spokesperson from ages 16-23. This mother then told me her son endured all variety of "micro-aggressions" from teachers and coaches afterward. My former classmate reported similar subtle retaliations after her mother had insisted she be allowed to graduate, despite her emotional challenges. These stories showed me the insidious ways faculty and staff had demonstrated willingness to make someone's life hell if they brought up reports of abuse at all.

~ ~ ~

In a follow up report to their investigation into private schools, the Boston Globe released a new article:

PRIVATE SCHOOLS, PAINFUL SECRETS

The unexpected price of reporting abuse: retaliation[13]

By Globe Staff July 20, 2016, 8:33 p.m.

The Globe Spotlight Team, in its ongoing investigation of abuses at New England private schools, found at least 15 instances of apparent retaliation against students who were sexually exploited by staffers or against employees who raised concerns about alleged sexual abuse and harassment. Some cases date back decades, while others are quite recent. But all of them are still raw for the people who felt the backlash...

The retribution, they say, came in various forms, including abusers lashing out at their accusers or enlisting other students to ostracize them, and administrators punishing or expelling students who complained of being victimized.

Marje Monroe, who said she previously faced reprisals for reporting alleged abuse at an independent school in Florida, has learned hard lessons about the culture of private schools.

"In a boarding community, especially, it is very painful to admit that someone you live with, raise your children with, and work with could betray your community," she said. "It becomes easier to blame the messenger for lying or causing the unease and tension."

~ ~ ~

[13] Globe Staff, July 20, 2016, https://www.bostonglobe.com/metro/2016/07/20/victims-abuse-private-schools-sometimes-face-retaliation-instead-sympathy/6SdTGZKxzkamgApl84NKHO/story.html

Whenever I hear someone refer to the "culture" of a place, I always return to the Anthropological definition of culture: "Behavior that is learned and shared". From another post on The Amends Project site:

What is a bystander?

In the MVP (Mentors in Violence Prevention) Model, a bystander is defined as a family member, friend, classmate, teammate, coworker—anyone who has a family, school, social, or professional relationship with someone who might in some way be abusive or experiencing abuse.

"Bystander" also refers to anyone in a wider peer culture, whether or not they are present at the time of a specific incident.

The goal is to help people move from being passive bystanders to empowered and active ones, and thus, change the social acceptability of harassment, abuse, or violence.

This really begs the question: What role do we each have to play? I have an ongoing hope that those who are standing-by (in very close range) shift from feelings of powerlessness ("I don't make decisions here") to empowerment: "I can shift the way culture happens here by even small acts of solidarity and resistance."

What does empower people in these moments?

We can all be agents of cultural change. For, what is learned can be un-learned. What is shared can be intentionally not shared, even while connection is preserved.

By good fortune, I soon found a group who was actively working to change the culture at these institutions around the country.

All Survivors Day

"Whatever you are ignoring is not going to go away.
Whatever you're ignoring is only going to get worse.
Whatever you're ignoring will be there
to be reckoned with until you reckon with it."

— Isabel Wilkerson

The suggestion that we organized alumni make ourselves a presence at Open House was getting real on social media. I'd already reached an uncomfortably low place in my personal resources. A family at my child's school miraculously reached out one day, to offer me their downstairs apartment at whatever I could afford. Blessings were many, yet this was all growing beyond what I could manage. I hesitated at the thought of traveling east again. Energy was still coursing through the group, while I tried to stay focused on The Justice CORPS Initiative and keeping a balance in my life. I had updated the model and proposed it to Lawrence Academy officials again on October 18. Once again, they declined.

One graduate shared her concerns that people were unlikely to come to Open House if I wasn't there. She saw me as a leader of this movement and doubted whether people could really have cohesion on this without me.

Fellow students started another GoFundMe fundraiser, and soon, another large donation appeared. Traveling started to feel possible. I made an Evite invitation to focus the energy around what that presence would look like. I sent it to about 90 former students and others following the effort. I composed a new letter for school leaders on "how to respond", first asking the most vocal people for feedback, and then sending.

The idea was, the school's "independent" investigation was not going to help them discover how to best respond, as Bruce MacNeil's words had stated. It was safe to say - this was not the goal of the investigation. They'd had information all along and still responded with denial and secrecy. The school was now being sued over Pete Regis, and the report would supplement their defenses in court.

~ ~ ~

Amidst all of this, I encountered a beautiful alignment in my research. SNAP, the Survivors Network of Those Abused by Priests was hosting a new event called All Survivors Day. It would be held on Saturday, November 3, 2018, just after All Saints Day on November 1 and All Souls Day, November 2.

November 3 was also the date of Lawrence Academy's Open House.

Demonstrations were being held around the country at schools, community centers, and places of worship. Organizers described All Survivors Day as:

"An international day to recognize survivors of sexual abuse, bring their stories into the light, raise awareness of the widespread nature of the issue and organize for change in the culture that allows sexual abuse to continue."

Now, I had to go.

Returns

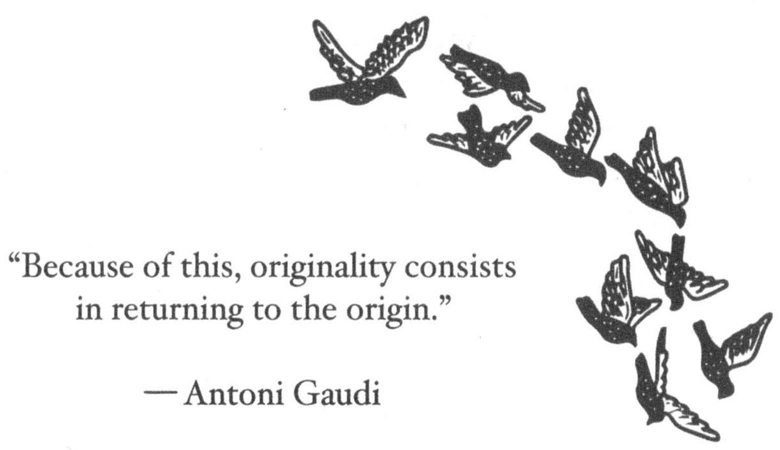

"Because of this, originality consists
in returning to the origin."

— Antoni Gaudi

Open House

"Throw your dreams into space like a kite,
and you do not know what it will bring back,
a new life, a new friend, a new love, a new country."

— Anais Nin

When I looked down on the city of Boston from the plane this time, it was with entirely new eyes.

I saw the ongoing problem of cover-up culture at Lawrence Academy of Groton, MA, and how it had transferred itself right onto new leadership. I returned to the east coast free of illusions. I saw the size and scope of Dan Scheibe's words (or had they all been written by Paul?) and I wasn't buying any of them. Now, their message and its delivery were so clearly unimpressive to me. All of their tactics looked appropriately small, in proportion to the urgency of what most needed to happen on a cultural level. The larger reality was too extraordinary, by contrast, around each of those moves.

These were unhealed men in an unhealed institution. Not only that, they were representatives of many who resisted the very thing that would free everyone connected to the painful legacy, if only they could let go.

I had felt the devastation along with every alumni or parent who reached out, being with people whose hearts - even while aching - were alive with the humane response to these incidents. The strength of their authenticity towered over the school's false statements like ancient redwoods over a withering patch of blackberry brambles.

~ ~ ~

The spirit of the road felt very near to me on this trip. I had to rely on a familiar kind of faith, too, since I was traveling to the east coast with only $218 available to me in cash or credit. I still had to get around, eat for three days, and make my stand where it mattered. What first looked to be a rally, with alumni in attendance while I held court on the quad, revealed itself to be an online show of rage for many. I didn't understand why. I count it among the mysteries of social media, which I choose to bypass. Where words don't line up with action, I'll just carry on in my own way.

So, I'd made the mental and emotional shifts on the plane heading east.

My childhood friend picked me up from Boston's Logan Airport in the wee hours, and we traveled to the home of my friend's brother outside the city. His family's carriage house would be my lodging. What a joy, having a long-time friend so close, reminding me of who I've always been, as I set forth to do something I'd never done.

Then, I found an email the following morning saying that Lawrence Academy staff had discovered news of our efforts. They were contacting All Survivors Day organizers to remove all information. Silencing returned, eclipsing the choice to stand in solidarity with survivors. It was a lost opportunity for integrity on their part. They acted again like people with something terrible to hide, and angry tensions were already mounting.

~ ~ ~

I now want to share what unfolded at Open House, as I wrote it by email to a dear friend in California. We met when I was 20 - a full twenty years earlier at that point - as neighbors in Eureka, California. Our closeness began when I was new to learning the adult world of rent payments, school, and job commitments. We share a great understanding and comfort.

Here you go:

I am amazed at how hard/sad it has been to be back [in Washington]. It was an AMAZING trip. Just every phase of it was meaningful and full of love and purpose.

When I flew out of Boston, I felt again all the sadness of how much I'd been compelled to run away at 17/18. How my leaving had been such a compulsion, and seeing all the connection that was lost. It was funny. I felt no angst about the east coast. Just a reminiscent sadness that it all went down that way.

So, it probably begins with the days leading up to flying. I'd sent that Evite, and soon realized I had zero yes responses.

What I got were quick No's from people who were either out of town or had some other quick answer. I got silence from everyone else.

This reality made a big difference in my plans. It was confusing - and still hurts a bit. So many people said things about standing with me, and 'we're coming for you!' (meaning headmaster), and more. Then, silence. It took some strength to reconcile this in my heart and soul. Folks were so vocal on social media. Did this not translate?

I decided, the night before my flight, I would have to go as an independent agent. Me plus 2-3 friends was not going to make a presence. I would register, attend programming, hand out info cards, and have many 1-on-1 conversations with prospective parents. I saw the beauty of this too!

So, I arrived at my friend's brother's beautiful carriage house outside Boston for the night. I got the privacy to sleep and gather my thoughts alone. I felt clear, focused.

Then, I got an email from someone at Lawrence Academy the morning of 11/2. They had found the listing for the event at www.allsurvivorsday.com. It was probably their investigators. I imagine they are regular visitors to the Amends Project site. I even have a new post planned to send just to them. If they're trolling me, I figure it's time I say hello directly!

So -- someone tipped them off that we planned to gather.

The email to the organizers was all huffy and hepped-up on fear. Ugh. What was great was that the organizers were so supportive of me and something happening. They asked, could you gather in front of the school? What if we change the address to Main Street & Powderhouse Road (the school has this very distinct little 'street' through campus).

So, I love that they didn't just acquiesce to the demands. They took the school name off and changed the location just enough to be legit. But it still screamed Lawrence Academy to anyone who looked. That was quite reassuring.

I consulted with Sybil — who was absolutely my right hand gal in all things! — and we debate some more about how I will register. There is a simple online form. We plan to have me sign in early that morning. Sybil gathers balloons, cardboard for signs, and clipboards (I'd written up a petition for parents to sign). All is prepared for the morning.

Saturday, I wake and learn the registration form is no longer active. Uh oh. So, I figure I'll register on-site. I want to be as thorough and legit as possible, so I can say, "I have every right to be here.", etc.

So I pack up and go. I decide to place the balloons and sign after I register, so as not to draw attention. I notice they have men (likely police + staff) in covered golf carts at both entrances. They are clearly patrolling the access points and ready to break up any gathering.

I park across from this church, tucked into the front of campus - that otherwise looks like part of the school if you don't know the finer details. This is where I saw the glorious sign, "If you want peace, work for justice.". I knew this was where I would have to make the visual statement. Both for resonance and the logistics of the sign being "off campus property".

~ ~ ~

So, I pull up to campus and park on the street in front of the church. I see the men in the cart. I figure, I'm in character. I wore a nice casual dress, boots, and my most professional-looking jacket. I'm just going to check out Open House. I walk past them (not right past, but the next driveway over), trembling a little but focused.

I fall in step with a group of people, which feels safer as I walk up the hill. Soon, I hear the head guy say, "Let's just duck in here and catch the program - we can register afterward.". I know that won't work for me, so I break away and head for the registration area.

Inside the building, two female students stand in welcome to the doors for the inner room to sign in. I see tables, A-L | M-Z | Walk-Ins. So, I go casually to the walk-ins table. I write my name on a sticker, and the woman starts to take down my name on her list. In retrospect, her hands were shaking terribly - which makes me wonder if she knew then who I was and was scared to be the one checking me in.

Clearly, by what unfolds, many had been told or warned about my coming.

But, I'm following protocol. I get my sticker and head toward the auditorium. As I leave the inner room, this African-American female student looks at me and says, "Are you a parent of a student?" and I say, "No, an alumna." Then, quickly, I ask, "Restrooms are over here?" and they nod. I walk on...

When I come out, I see this young woman whispering and looking all suspicious toward me beside an old, male teacher. They approach. The man says, "Vanessa" (he remembers me) and I say, "Rob, you've aged well if you don't mind my saying..."

"What are you doing on campus?"

"Just here to attend Open House programming."

"With any others?"

"No"

He looks ay my face suspiciously for a while as the moment lingers. I stay calm and give off an air of, *'What? I'm just here to attend'*. And I am.

I walk on down to the auditorium.

It's packed - and I have checked in about ten minutes past 9 am. That was fairly intentional. I soon find a seat along an aisle. It's fucking odd to be there. All the hopeful looking parents and early teens. Open House is the biggest self-promotion event of the whole year. This is where they serve all the bullshit to give a certain impression. It does, admittedly, become painful to watch.

Oh, interestingly, as I walk in, a woman looks right at me and says, "Hi Vanessa" in a calm, easy voice. It's Libby, the Assistant Head of Student Life - same young (my age?!) woman who sat in on the Restorative Justice Circle. She is very submissive to the headmaster. But I swear by reading her tone and body language that she is secretly proud of me for sticking with all of this. I know on some level, she wants to see a woman stand up to this - and her casual warmth toward me betrays her position. She seems glad or impressed that I've made it.

Pretty soon after I sit down, they decide to break the group in half. So, "If you have a blue folder, please file out and toward the Ansin Academic Center. You'll come back later for the panel. If you have a red folder (me), please get up and move toward the front of the theatre.

I do. This is where I start to feel it in my body. I am weak and worry that I won't stay standing. I decide I need to get pretty close to the front and center. I want the headmaster to see me clearly. I want to be 'in his face' and communicating nonverbally.

This all happens. Again, it is painful to see Dan Scheibe and associates brag about how great they are. He says things that are surreal in their untruth. Maybe they have held some truth at some time - but knowing their corrupt underbelly, they are glaring falsehoods to me. I don't clap at any of their speeches. I make consistent eye contact. I see the headmaster sweating a bit.

He even tells a story about meeting up with a male alumna twenty years later to hear about his life. The headmaster says, "This ethic of care, it's a generational thing.".

Wow. It is so fucking odd.

Then, we are finally excused. The part I was waiting for - the chance to mingle with prospective families - arrives.

As I get up, a teacher approaches me - she was there when I was a student. She starts chatting in a way that mocks the reality of the situation; of course she knows my engagement with the school. "How are you? What are you doing for work now?". I am not willing to bullshit.
"The thing with the school has been hard... I don't want to get into it. I'm feeling a bit rattled - all of what was said up there doesn't hold. But thanks for saying hi." I keep walking. It seems that stalling me with BS is one tactic.

Luckily, I then start making progress amidst the crowd. I approach a trio of two parents with a teen and ask, "Are you a prospective family?" They say yes. I say, "I'm a former student" (swoon or intrigue), "I'm working on positive change at the school," and hand them a card. I probably get to about five or six families.

One, in particular, asks, "How did you like it?" and I calmly say, "Some good, some not so good" (with a dead-pan sincerity) "I'm working on positive change at the school."

I do like to think I may have reached and spared some people. I brought an important level of awareness.

~ ~ ~

Then, while inside, right as I engage a mother, this older woman gets between us and says, "You can't be doing that." And I start right in with, "Don't interrupt me, that's rude, I was just talking to this mother." She tries again. Then, I look her calm in the face and say, "I have every right to be here. I am a former student. I registered. I am allowed to speak about my experience." Then, the prophetic moment - I breathe deep into my belly and say, "I'm here because I care."

I can tell she feels the truth of it and leaves me be. I don't like feeling her behind me, so I double back to walk the other way. I probably reach two more families.

Then, I step out of the building and decide to go peer over toward Main Street, to see if anyone has gathered. I don't see anyone. I start to walk into the building with the student mailboxes. I figure I will put a card in each kid's mailbox. But first, I see a sign over the stairs that says, "We cannot solve the problems we have today with the same mindset that created them." You know - the Einstein quote!

Funny, I'd used this in regards to the project. So, I start to tuck a card in beside it.

But then, the same African-American student comes in and says, "You can't do that." She had followed me in there. I concede and say, "Ok, I can see that.". She then says, "This building isn't part of Open House. Do you need a tour?" and I say, "No, I went here, so I know the campus." "Well, you have to leave this building," which strikes me as odd. If a parent wandered in, would they get that?

I say, "I want to know what they told you about me." (She is clearly handling me like a criminal, so I figure there had to be some fear-based propaganda). She says, "I don't feel at liberty to tell you that." To which I say, "They got you with silencing too, huh?". I feel disgusted by what this means about school leaders.

I later reflect on how exploitive it is to ask a minority female student to join your exclusion army. I can't stop seeing the obvious irony: I am on campus advocating for a systemic overhaul that would bring improved protections to minority students. In response, school leaders have enlisted a minority student to stop me, and essentially protect the status quo on their behalf. Did they get parent permission for that? Isn't that an ethical violation? Sybil is also later disgusted. She says, "It's one thing to get your staff to do shit like that - but, *kids*?!"

So, I walk out of the building, up toward the center of campus, with her trailing close behind me.

Here, it gets intense.

Heading right toward me on the one path are two police officers on either side of the woman who encountered me in the crowd. They are coming for me. In that moment, I think I have a tiny inkling of what soldiers must feel during warfare. Only, it's just me. I am unarmed. They are many.

They approach. Two officers (an African-American man and a caucasian female, maybe in her late 30s). One says, "You have to leave."

"I have every right to be here. I have registered. I am following all of your protocol and limits."

Another says, "You were going to have a gathering of people here."

"I cancelled that to stay within your limits.", I say.

"You're handing out materials."

"That isn't illegal," I point out. "If a parent is talking to another parent, and one is an insurance agent and the other needs insurance, they might exchange cards."

He counters, "But people aren't doing that."

"But they could if the moment arose," I point out. "It still isn't illegal."

"You have to leave."

"No, I don't."

This goes on for a little bit. I hold my ground. I am not breaking any laws. I know this.

Soon, the African-American man says, "Well, it's too late. You've already past a limit."

"If you don't want me to hand out information, just set the limit, and I'll respect it." I catch the hypocrisy and add, "How can I respect a limit if I don't know it?" Again, "You set a limit, and I'll respect it - but I do not have to leave campus."

Then he says, "If you don't leave, we'll arrest you for trespassing." Some more back and forth, and then I shift, "How do you feel that *This* is the response to a former student coming back to be on campus? What does that say about the school?"

The female officer speaks, "I'm just doing my job." Right. The futile cry of every wrong-doer in authority. Then, I finally address the older woman between them. She's not a cop.

"How do *You* feel that this is the response of the school to a former student?"

She has no significant answer but seems shaken out of the intensity enough to finally see how absurd this is.

The man continues, "If you don't leave, we have to arrest you for trespassing."

"What's that like?"

"I arrest you."

"No, I mean, how does that look? What's the process?" (clearly, considering it, as an option).

He clarifies, "I put you in handcuffs and walk you off campus."

Now, if I had someone to take a photo of that, I might have gone that route. If I could have utilized the moment to demonstrate how Fucking Ridiculous they are being about all of this, I would have. But, I had no photographer.

Still, they seem unnerved that I don't flinch at the suggestion. The male officer says, "I'm asking you to leave."

"But you're just the police - you can't ask me to leave a place."

Pause.

"I want to talk to the person that's asking me to leave. Bring them to me.", I continue.

Here, it starts to shift. The same female staff person then steps forward and says, "I'm the one. I'm asking you to leave."

There is a moment of breathing while I just stare at her. She soon says, "I'll talk to you." Pause again, as the energy shifts. "Let's take a walk," she offers.

I say, "Not if you are going to walk me off campus."

She says, "No, we'll just walk."

Then, the police turn and fall away. The battle has ended, and I am still standing. The staff woman and I start walking on campus, just the two of us.

I know, breathe in. Breathe out.

~ ~ ~

Consider for a moment here - many players are represented - except for the white male. Who is doing the protecting, and what is being protected? This moment of rising tension plays out in a mostly-white woman, a middle-aged white woman, a male police officer of color, a white woman police officer, and also a young woman of color, a student. The only persona not engaged in this showdown is the white male - for whom all privilege and protection flow to benefit.

Notice the players present and those absent from this showdown. What does it all say?

~ ~ ~

My email story continues.

She introduces herself, tells me her name is Jamie Baker and offers a hand. I don't shake it then. But we keep walking. I like to think she's just a little intimidated by watching me hold my ground like that. I remember now there was something in her face in that moment.

I ask again if she is going to escort me off campus. She says, "No, I'll follow your lead. We can go wherever you want to go."

Then, we set in to strolling. I start to tell her my story.

I'm hot from the stress of confrontation, so I hold my jackets in my arms, with just gloves on my hands. Naked arms in my short-sleeved dress. My system is slowly cooling down. It's very lightly raining, but I feel refreshed by this.

Soon, the same African-American student approaches us as we walk and hands us an open umbrella. I am confused and unsure of how to interpret this. I'd like to think it's pure compassion or humanity, but somehow it doesn't read that way. I start to wonder how many parents might have witnessed the showdown on the quad. That is the very center of campus.

As we walk, I tell her how I confronted Pete Regis ("at 16?!" she exclaims with pride). I get to point to the very dorm room where I shuddered in fear as he stalked me - a potent way to tell a story - right where it happened. We look up at that window together.

We walk and walk. I tell Jamie Baker about the Justice CORPS, about parents reaching out to me. She listens well. She asks if I think my seeking restitution for the past is muddying my efforts for change in the future. We revisit this point a few times.

Once alone, we clearly have a growing respect for each other. Turns out, she is the brand new Assistant Head for Academic Life. Technically speaking, the highest position under the headmaster. The other gal is more like a secretary to the headmaster (the woman who was warm and easy, and nearly happy to see me on campus again). This woman I am walking with has clout.

I end up spending over two hours with her. She invites me into her home, an old, white Colonial building on campus. I'd never been inside one of those staff houses. They're awfully nice. I take off my boots and my socks since they'd gotten soaked through with the rain. She starts to make tea, and I end up stepping with my bare feet onto something that I first think is a mushroom. Then, I see it's poop. She has an elderly dog, and it has left a pile of soft brown beside her kitchen table. What are the chances?!

This (as I'm not all too scared of poop, either, and react very calmly) also serves to humanize us more. I mean, she almost tried to kick me off campus. She watches me stand up to the police. We connect while walking through the drizzling rain. Then, I'm scrubbing dog poop off my bare feet in her kitchen - quite the emotional ground to cover in two hours.

We talk about the situation with the school. Jamie tells me about a psychologist she likes to read who writes on polarity theory. We even open to a page in her book with a diagram that illustrates personal responsibility within community responsibility. We marvel at the chances.

We like each other. We respect each other's minds. She starts to feel more like a colleague. I tell her I'm 40. She tells me she's 56. She is from Nashville, Tennessee. I tell her about my Grandad and the deep family roots in Chattanooga. She has been on the job only nine weeks; they recruited her to the position. The fact that she is new - and from a different region - gives me great hope in the possibility of someone with clear sight grasping the scope of this issue.

She explains that part of her job is making sure schools are living their missions in action. So, if a school's motto is, "Lawrence Academy inspires you to take responsibility for who you want to become... by calling on each other to engage in a plurality of perspectives...", Jamie looks at the data to ask, how is the school living that value in practice? It needs to be quantifiable and measurable.

At times, she offers me guidance or mentoring. At times, I'm just filling her in. She tells me about an upcoming accreditation conference. I tell her how strangely unreceptive and even aggressive the guy who oversees this school's accreditation became over The Justice CORPS. I speculate that he's too much in it. He knows Steve Hahn (former headmaster) and was headmaster at Tabor Academy in Marion, Massachusetts until 2012.

I don't talk of it at the time, but this man was featured in a Boston.com article titled, "New England Boarding School Heads are Making Bank"[14] as having *the* highest pay of any headmaster in the region at the time ($822,011/year in 2012; a full $118,000 *higher* than the second-ranked headmaster). How does one person get away with that kind of money and

14 Megan Turchi, Boston.com June 24, 2014, https://www.boston.com/news/local-news/2014/06/23/new-england-boarding-school-heads-are-making-bank

become that reactive about an oversight body?

Anyway, soon, Open House is ending, and Jamie has a 12:30 meeting. I'm wiped-out from the exhaustion of facing the squad - and the fact that I couldn't even eat that morning.

We say goodbye. On the way out, she says, "Maybe we met for a reason."

I agree.

It very much has that feeling - especially with how thrilled she is over the Justice CORPS model. She wants to see it take. She kept saying this school was "too sunburned" and may not be willing now. She is encouraging me to take the model elsewhere for a pilot.

At this point, I just can't imagine devoting any energy to this without being well-paid. I also struggle with the idea of an immune system kicking in - only to be redirected to places where disease may not be festering.

~ ~ ~

After our talk, I decide I still need to place the balloons and the sign and snap that picture. It is a valuable awareness-raising tool. So, I do that. I'm still rattled (mostly tired and hungry at that point). The police at the entrances are gone - so none see me directly. Still, faculty and staff are crawling all over the place.

I get the photos.

I start to drive away from Main Street/campus. Then, I revive enough to try stopping into a roadside deli, to see if they'll let me put a stack of cards on their counter. This experience was amazing, too.

I stand in line to wait to ask the question. The man gestures to me, the way New Englanders do, to say directly, "What do you want?". I call out in response, from behind someone ordering. I say, "I have these info cards, and wondered if you could set them out somewhere." Right after this, a man approaches me and asks, "Can I see one?" I hand him one. Even without his seeing the back - so just looking at "The Amends Project" and the logo, he

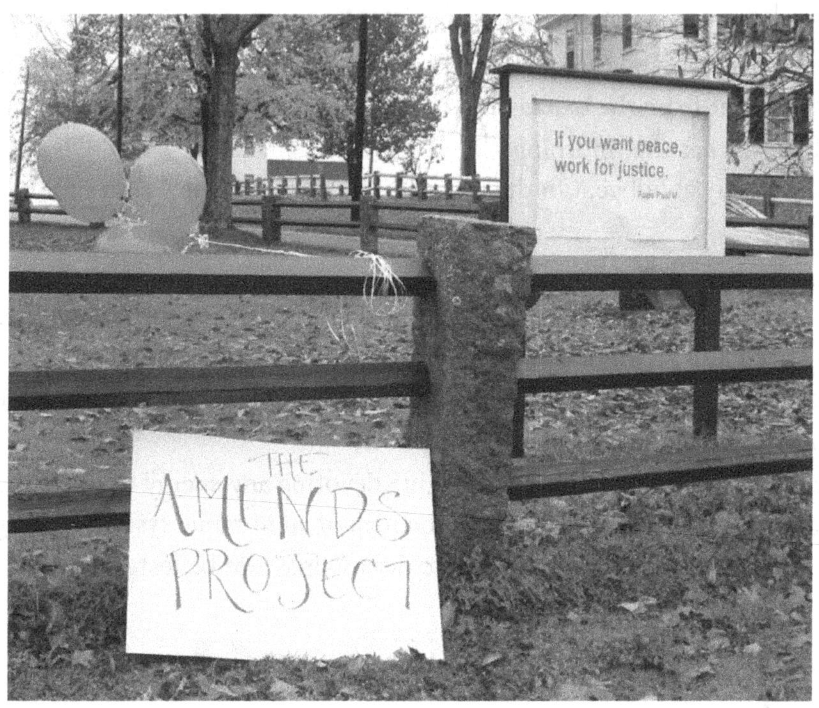

looks at me, smiles, and says, "My wife was also a survivor." He is nodding approvingly. It kind of blows me away that 1. He either guesses what this is or recognizes it! 2. He is so plainly supportive - no controversy with everyday folks.

I realize soon, people OUTSIDE the school are all in support of this. Of course! They co-exist with the elitists in a rural town, and yet, they know what's up. I am heartened to no longer be "the enemy" and, instead, met with such honest, grateful support. They happily take a stack.

This emboldens me to drive back toward campus and hit the strip of businesses right across from the school. It includes "GroHo's" The Groton House of Pizza, where we all used to hang out after school. I start with an upscale flower shop. They look at the cards, flip it over - where it says, "Seeking Lasting, Positive Change! Lawrence Academy has a cover-up problem. We're here to help." She looks. Says nothing, but calmly accepts and places them right in front of the register.

This happens over and over and over again. Only an Asian woman at a dry cleaners turns me down - and she may have just been confused - I notice they didn't have any materials out at all. The pizza house seems to have the Very Same guy who worked there back in the day. A family member of his was the first to thank me for my efforts. Back when I was 16, she told me, "I'm so glad you did that (confronted Pete) because he did the same things to me when I was your age."

So, there I stand at 40. I swear it's the same man. He looks to be just near 50. I can easily see now that he was only around ten years older than us. I worry he'll recognize me as easily. Yet, he says nothing directly. He reads the card and says, "Lawrence Academy, huh?" in a slightly bitter, sarcastic tone. They got A LOT of business from the kids at the school. He paused and said, "Put them right over there." Total support.

I have to tell you - most moving to me was an older man named Gary, of Gary's Farm Stand. This place has been in operation forever. I don't know how long. I walked in thinking, "Ok, a wholesome rural farm stand - maybe not my best bet...". Still, I had to try. There are only so many businesses surrounding the school. He's the only one in there, a spacious barn-shaped storefront. I stand waiting a while by the counter until he emerges from somewhere in back. A slow-moving, but strong old man.

I show him what I have. He looks at it. He reads the Lawrence Academy part and points to a picture on his wall of a pretty young woman (likely a professional 'senior portrait' photograph). He says, "My granddaughter went there [he says her name, which I already forget]. Do you recognize her name?" I say I don't. He continues reading...

"Cover-ups, huh?" He pauses. "What are they covering up?" I look at him directly and say, "child abuse." Then, he gets so focused; it nearly makes me cry. I was incredibly moved.

He takes the stack and balances it right against his register. He has nothing like that in the farm stand. Then, he says, "Let's put one on the door, too." So, I walk with him over to his double glass doors - an In door and an Out door. Both clear glass. The sincerity in his dark blue eyes was profound. He very slowly tapes one of my business cards right at eye level on the entry door. I help smooth the tape. Then, he says, "Let's put one over here, too." We start to tape one to the Out door.

He was just so determined and un-self-conscious about making this very clear statement on his store front. Taping my little business cards to the empty glass doors. I asked his name and he said, "Gary", which is how I realized he is The Gary, of the long-time farm stand.

He just seemed to communicate so much in his eyes. I read, "This is so absolutely important, there is no question that we need to do everything we can. I don't care what any of my customers might think." He was resolute, and I was deeply moved.

I got a few more farm stands and shops and soon was nearly out of cards.

~ ~ ~

I went and got groceries. I visited Nagog Hill - the magical place I lived in 2006 when I spent the year back east. I caught my breath. It was around 2 pm. I then knew it was important to update the Amends Project homepage - to reflect a new message directly for those seeing the cards. So, I went to the library with my laptop.

Soon, I was completely exhausted.

I had considered other moves but started to rethink my plan. Most of all, I recognized a limit with what my body could do. Yes, I held my ground to the police pretty easily, but it left me tired (after traveling so far) in a way like crying does - a deep, undeniable exhaustion. I knew it was best to get back to Sybil's by dark and eat a good meal with a great friend. So, that's what I did.

We had so much fun. I got to meet her new, ideal partner. They are so well-matched! I talked a little about the day - but left most of the processing for when Sybil and I would have a walk together in the morning. We just laughed and enjoyed and drank and ate.

It was AMAZING. All of it.

Again, not what I pictured. And yes, I am sifting through odd feelings about alumni not actually showing. Though, I did feel compassion for how much harder it would be to do all of this at close range.

The distance (of the whole country) not only gives me perspective - but also freedom. In my day-to-day, I am free from the weight of the school leaders' presence. I don't feel their hypocrisies and pressures as I move through my life. I do see how tough it would be to be *in it* and confronting them.

I remain glad to be the one to do it.

Balancing That Story

By the spring of 2019, I'd had video conference meetings with leaders of both The Association of Boarding Schools (TABS) and The National Association of Independent Schools (NAIS). True, I had an unresolved conflict with one school. I sensed that old trepidation of others to get involved. Yet, by this point, I believe my endurance, over years without any settlement, was proving that my commitment to positive change was the priority.

Each had sat on the Task Force on Educator Sexual Misconduct, established in 2016, to create Guidelines for an appropriate response to these situations. It was a devoted effort. Their goal was "to contribute to a broader understanding of educator sexual misconduct in independent schools and to identify specific strategies that independent schools can take to prevent and respond to misconduct effectively". Along with fourteen others, these two leaders contributed to a draft document. They opened this up for review by professionals over the course of two years. Then, in 2018, the Task Force released the final guidelines, called "Prevention & Response: Recommendations for Independent School Leaders".[15]

I noticed this line as I read, "*Schools that honestly and openly confront abuse are the standard-bearers for the independent school community.*". Valuable as they were, I realized these were static guidelines only. I had similarly

[15] TABS & NAIS, 2018, https://www.nais.org/media/Nais/Articles/Documents/Prevention-and-Response-Task-Force-Report-2018.pdf

learned (in my conversations with New England Association of Schools and Colleges Accreditation Director, Jay Stroud, former headmaster of Tabor Academy) that Accreditation is very simply a statement of intentions.

There was clearly a missing piece - in measuring whether these guidelines were met or fulfilled. One more step to follow through to positive change. Who was watching to see that all schools met these standards? There were standards for academics, sports, and other criteria in an accreditation process. Yet, not one for student safety. My Justice CORPS model brought enforcement and accountability to their work in creating recommendations. So, I contacted TABS and NAIS to share news of my work.

They were naturally concerned and eager to see new solutions.

Massachusetts State Representatives expressed their interest, too. A few said they would consider giving their endorsement (as I'd been asking many to do) after a pilot run of the program. Once I filed Articles of Incorporation to make The Amends Project a state nonprofit, I started applying for grants to help see me through to getting that pilot up and running.

It was Pete Upham, at TABS, who suggested that I give The Amends Project a more official structure. He explained that it would open up possibilities for how we could intersect as organizations. Donna Orem and Myra McGovern at NAIS offered the suggestion of a Seal of Excellence in Child Safety for participating schools that reached new levels of quality response.

With encouragement from a great colleague, Shael Norris of Safe BAE, I filed articles of incorporation, establishing my second nonprofit.

~ ~ ~

Along the way, I also had the great fortune to find Mike Rinaldi. Mike became my latest Advisor to The Amends Project, bringing immense kindness, courage, and dedication. As Assistant Principal at Stamford High School in Stamford, Connecticut, he and his colleagues reported the school's

Principal for covering up sexual abuse of a student by a teacher. The subsequent response of the Superintendent and the Board of Education compelled him to speak up, repeatedly, about what he saw as a highly unethical practice. He, along with Terri Miller of SESAME, Stop Educator Sexual Abuse Misconduct and Exploitation, devoted persistent, heroic energy to stopping what people commonly referred to as "passing the trash".

This is the other cowardly, "not dealing with it" response, where an employee who commits abuse is simply moved to a new school, district, or parish (in the case of priests). Often, they leave with glowing recommendations and even generous severance packages. Remember, even a documented child-molester-groundskeeper got health insurance for life from Lawrence Academy of Groton, Massachusetts, on his way out, before my speech in 2001.

Mike kept speaking out, attending meetings to address the school board, challenging his colleagues - going to work alongside them every day - until he got results. Because of the precedent he helped to set, the practice is now illegal in his home state of Connecticut.

~ ~ ~

These same patterns have played out in churches and schools across the country. The connection, of course, is that men in established institutions have been abusing their power. Where people have believed priests held the keys to the afterlife, they believed headmasters held the keys to the good life.

Over what people wanted for their souls, they believed priests had exclusive dominion. For what they wanted for their kids, they believed headmasters were the gatekeepers. It is the perception that priests and headmasters are exploiting. It's worth considering, then, that neither is true. Perhaps, heaven is only as close as our integrity and choosing love. Success is as accessible as living your passion prosperously, among a network of healthy connections.

During one of our conversations, Mike pointed out the unique challenge I faced in bringing positive change to private schools. "People are used to complaining to the state [which oversees public schooling] because it all comes from our taxes and is governed by elected officials. When you point this out to parents in private schools, it's like you're saying, 'Hey, that $60,000 you spent this year was a mistake'. They may see it as a criticism of their own judgment. I mean, we all want to believe we're making the right choices for our kids.".

This is true. It must be embarrassing, on top of everything else, to have to admit you were duped by a glossy catalog, and your investment is not what you thought. One woman on the other side of the country is far easier to critique than a whole community you bought into with your time, money, and your precious child.

Mike's story is the closest I have to a model for achieving what I have set out to do. I value him and his counsel immensely. He had the conviction to challenge his co-workers in real-time, risking far more than social awkwardness. He suffered retaliation for speaking out initially. Yet, he endured. Then, with these changes in place, the School Board unanimously voted to appoint him Principal of Connecticut's Westhill High School. Mike Rinaldi has truly earned the role of authority in the best possible way.

~ ~ ~

I'd been begging Rick Sobey to write a follow up article about The Justice CORPS for months. It had been seven months since the defamation piece following the Public Response Event back in summer 2018. That had been the last word on the matter in the Lowell Sun. That would not do - not after all I'd given to the larger mission.

With Articles of Incorporation, I had another reason to pester him to give me that piece. Rick had moved over to The Boston Herald, no doubt, his coverage of this story giving him credibility to advance in his own career. I did not let up.

Finally, April 2, 2019, we got it out to the greater Boston area:

NEWS

Justice CORPS initiative aims to empower school abuse victims[16]

By **BOSTON HERALD**
PUBLISHED: April 2, 2019 at 12:00 a.m. I UPDATED: September 10, 2019 at 1:51 p.m.

GROTON — Critics of transparency at boarding schools and other educational institutions have glared at the child abuse loophole for decades. After receiving a report of abuse on their campus, officials decide whether the school should investigate the alleged abuse or if police should get involved, the critics emphasize.

Far too often, this policy has allowed schools to cover-up scandals involving school personnel, according to advocates who want this protocol overhauled and the loophole closed.

One of these champions for change is Vanessa (Fadjo) Osage, who last year told The Sun about a former Lawrence Academy groundskeeper sexually molesting her in the 1990s, when she was 14 years old.

Osage is now moving forward with a proposal, the Justice CORPS Initiative, that she says would empower students and gives families the right to decide how abuse matters are handled — ensuring abuse is not swept under the rug by school leaders.

Preventing abuse and cover-ups at schools has been her mission for the last 25 years, she stressed.

---

[16] Rick Sobey, The Boston Herald, April 2, 2019, https://theamendsproject.com/press/

"We need to resolve the cover-up problem once-and-for-all," said Osage, who now lives in Washington state. "This structure would bring about positive change in schools."

She has submitted the Justice CORPS Initiative to Lawrence Academy multiple times in the last year.

The latest 9-page iteration of the proposal, evolved with the help of professionals in education and child abuse prevention around the country, was sent to the school last month.

It has been radio silence from the school, Osage said.

"They say they don't need this, but this is still a very pressing need there," she said of Lawrence Academy.

A Lawrence Academy spokesman declined to respond to questions about Osage and the Justice CORPS Initiative.

Osage's proposal would bring together a group of non-affiliated adults who act as a volunteer oversight board — receiving and reporting on abuse incidents at the school.

The school year would begin with an assembly to introduce the Justice CORPS members and train students, faculty and staff on expectations for behavior, how to report abuse, and what happens following reports of abuse. Students would be able to anonymously report the incidents to the Justice CORPS. There would be a monthly recording of incident reports, incidents verified, and a score of the responses enacted by school officials. The annual report would be available for public review.

"The school doesn't get to intercept that loop," Osage said. "It becomes an honest record of abuse, a true record of how well schools are responding to abuse."

One of the goals is to ultimately decrease the incidence of child abuse on high school campuses by 50 percent or more, in three-year cycles, until there is none, Osage said.

The Justice CORPS Initiative is a proposal through The Amends Project, which Osage started online. Last week, she filed articles of incorporation for The Amends Project to be a registered nonprofit in Washington.

She's now seeking grants to get the Justice CORPS funded, and launch a pilot program for the 2019/2020 school year.
"I'm highly motivated to get things in place and move forward with this by May," Osage said.

Their Report & Mine

"It's important for institutions to be careful
about the word 'independent'
and be transparent about what this means...
They are paying for these services,
it's not like these are volunteers coming in."

— Paul G. Lannon Jr., partner at Holland & Knight,
attorney for Lawrence Academy of Groton, MA
as quoted in the New York Times, September 28, 2017

Dan Scheibe had sent a message to their list on July 26, 2018:

"The school, under the authorization of the Board of Trustees, has engaged Sanghavi Law Office to perform an independent investigation into reports or allegations involving Mr. Regis. Elizabeth Sanghavi and Kate Upham from Sanghavi Law Office will be conducting this investigation.

"We strongly encourage participation and cooperation with this investigation. The more information Lawrence Academy has, the more effective we can be in responding to alumni who may have experienced misconduct while here and in protecting current and future students."

Concerned about the contradictions, I'd contacted Paul Lannon for clarification after returning from Open House. First, in November, I left a voicemail, to which I received a lengthy email reply.

Mon, Nov 12, 2018, 8:57 AM

Dear Vanessa,

With respect to the investigation, please bear in mind three key features: external, independent and experienced. Given that the school's own conduct is at issue, the current administration, with the knowledge and approval of the Board of Trustees, decided to hire an *external* investigator -- someone not employed by or affiliated with the school -- to provide an objective perspective. The school wants someone who can step back and provide an outsider's view; someone who can be candid with the school about what went wrong as well as what may have been handled appropriately.

...The pending investigation by Sanghavi Law Office is the best opportunity available to *uncover and share* the facts about abuse by Mr. Regis as well as the school's response. I encourage you again to be part of this important process. The information you share will make a difference. Your story is at the heart of this matter.

...I hope you will take full advantage of this opportunity.

I wanted to address sooner than later your concerns about the investigation because your participation would greatly benefit other victims, other students, and the whole school community.

Sincerely,

Paul

Paul actually tried to appeal to my urge for positive impact, to convince me to add to their version of the story.

Nov 15, 2018, 8:03 AM

Paul,

I find this all contradictory and misleading.

Remember, I have become the outsider with the perspective to candidly see what has gone wrong at the school. I have had that perspective for 25 years. People have been sharing similar stories with me all that time; I continue to receive stories families would not currently trust the school (or investigators) to hold. Therefore, I am more experienced - and also less biased - than investigators hired to create a report.

If your goal is to complete that report - then, it is in your best interest to advise the school leaders to accept my proposals today.

ONLY then will I participate in the investigation.

Acceptance in the Justice CORPS, and the good faith gesture of *finally* doing right by me is, in fact, the step that would most benefit other victims, other students and the school community.

This petition also gives me assurance that this is true.

I look forward to seeing those documents, signed & notarized [settlement and agreement to participate in The Justice CORPS]. Let me know if you have any questions. I will accept copies scanned by email, followed by paper copies in the mail.

PO Box 1559
Bellingham, WA 98227

Thank you,

Vanessa Osage

Weeks went by, with no response or confirmation. I also discovered that Elizabeth Sanghavi is a former associate of Holland & Knight, the law firm currently representing the school. This cancelled out his "not affiliated with the school" statement. It added to the irony that, according to the New York Times article, the school would be hiring the firm at up to $2 million in compensation. With no reason to believe the report would be unedited, I asked Paul to back up his words with documentation.

Sat, Dec 22, 2018, 11:29 AM

Paul,

You have said that the investigation will be presented and available in full, unedited form to the public.

To verify your word, please send scanned copy of the signed agreement between school officials and Sanghavi Group.

Thank you,

Vanessa

Paul,

I ask politely, again, for verification that findings from the investigation will not be edited, abbreviated or altered by the school. Additionally, any agreement about the scope of investigation (whether of actions by school officials or a former employee) is highly relevant.

As we learned in **the New York Time article**[17], where you yourself were quoted as questioning how truly "independent" these investigations are, these parameters make or break the believability of such reports.

"But critics say that the firms, often described by administrators as "independent," can be too close to the schools they are investigating. Ultimately, it is the schools that pay their bills, and decide what information will be released.

"If they do this full time, there is a perception issue, that they're not going to draw tough conclusions in all cases," said Roderick MacLeish, a lawyer who represents victims of abuse at private schools. "If you're going to keep doing this, how tough are you going to be on some private school client, when you are basically marketing yourself for other investigations in the future?"

Even the firms that conduct them acknowledge that the investigations are not free of conflict.

"It's important for institutions to be careful about the word 'independent' and be transparent about what this means," said **Paul G. Lannon Jr.**, *a partner at Holland & Knight [attorney for Lawrence Academy of Groton, MA]. "They are paying for these services, it's not like these are volunteers coming in."*

"...At the outset, schools generally outline parameters for the firms they hire. Some ask investigators to focus on a specific span of time, or on adult misconduct, as opposed to student-on-student sexual violence. They will decide whether the inquiry will culminate in a written report, or some kind of oral presentation. A budget is discussed. Some reports name several perpetrators and the administrators who protected them, while others present almost no information about what happened.

Some pledge ahead of time to release their findings, while others wait to see what is uncovered before they decide what they will make public."

---

17 Staff Writer, The New York Times, September 28, 2017, https://www.nytimes.com/2017/09/28/nyregion/lawyers-prep-school-sexual-abuse.html

If I do not receive this verification by **Monday April 15, 2019**, I will conclude that all findings will be subject to the school's discretion; and I will proceed accordingly.

Thank You,

Vanessa Osage

Wed, Dec 26, 2018, 2:31 PM

Paul,

Please also send scanned signed copies of agreements that outline the scope of the investigation.

Thank you,

Vanessa

I called Paul Lannon at his Boston office for the first time while awaiting this clarification. He answered, and we did talk for over thirty minutes. He hung up in frustration first. It would be the one and only time Paul would take my call. During our talk, I asked, "Why would you *not* encourage school leaders to accept The Justice CORPS as part of settlement?". He responded with an immediate, shrill alarm in his voice, "I would lose my job!"

I'll let you draw whatever conclusion you will from that stance.

The more time passed, the more it became clear that the alliance of Sanghavi Group, Paul Lannon and Lawrence Academy would produce a highly subjective result. They were starting with a hypothesis: Pete Regis was wrong, yet school leaders were essentially innocent and absolved. The parties formed this alliance to produce research to a specific end. "*Come to us with your information,*"the clarion call rang, "*so we can tell everyone how it is.*" the subtext echoed out indefinitely.

Also, from the New York Times article, with direct mention of Sanghavi Group, hired by Lawrence Academy in 2018:

"The Sanghavi Law Office, a Massachusetts firm founded by a former civil rights lawyer at the United States Education Department, has conducted investigations at a number of schools, including Phillips Academy in Andover. The school released a letter to its community last year with some findings, and then in July, it released the full report, which named perpetrators *but provided few hints about what administrators knew or what they did with the information they had.*"

~ ~ ~

It was April before I heard from Paul Lannon again. Nearly four months had passed.

Apr 11, 2019, 1:31 PM

Hi Vanessa,

I spoke with the school about your questions below. I can confirm that yes*, at the time the investigators' report is released publicly the school and the investigators will also be addressing publicly the scope of the investigation and the nature of the engagement. I don't have further information to share at this time.

Sincerely,

Paul

'We'll release what we want to release when we are ready. We have that control'...

I kept a record of this effort to "hold leaders accountable" on The Amends Project website. I wrote:

* Note, if **Accountability** seeks answers, it is also astute enough to recognize whether or not a question has been truly answered.

There was not a yes/no question in my original message to Paul. If there was, the answer would be, "No, we will not provide any verification."

I did not ask the question, "Will the school retain control of all information – including the scope of investigation and the level of disclosure with Sanghavi Group – until they can orchestrate a precise release when it best suits them?" To this question, the answer would be 'yes'.

2:19 AM

Thank you, Paul,

I am interpreting this vagueness to mean (as was confirmed to fellow alumni by phone) the investigation has only focused on the actions of former employee, Peter Regis.

I also conclude that the school has retained the right to control the contents of the report, so that findings will be released only according to their interests.

I will have more for you by Monday.

I later asked when they would release the report, and they would not give me that information. But, I did get a call from Dan Scheibe in April, on the eve of the report's release.

~ ~ ~

They had arranged the conversation by email a few days prior. Dan Scheibe had asked if we could speak on a Wednesday. They would be releasing their report on Thursday.

I called Noah and talked to him about it. Since they were going to expose what they deemed appropriate, all my fight hackles were raised.

He was hopeful. He said, "It may be in their best interest to do right by you at this point. They know you have the other side of the story. Maybe it's good news they want to share with you."

He had other guidance for me, as well, about letting Dan do all the talking. "Just see why they are reaching out", he urged. I promised to follow up with him afterward. I'd been in touch with a few new attorneys around Boston after the August 2018 defamation in The Lowell Sun. I understood my strengthening legal position. Dan Scheibe, through Paul's counsel, was racking up more and more legal charges - not from the 1990s - but in modern-day. No statute of limitations required.

I only had twenty minutes and let Dan know my time would be tight. He was very slow and measured as we spoke - obviously building up to something. He referenced some of the *"the school could have done more"* language. He seemed to expect gushing or gratitude from me. I stayed firm while awaiting whatever was clearly coming.

Then, he said, "We contacted your father to get a statement.". I instantly roared, "That's my father, Dan Scheibe.". I struggled to contain my rage. "You agreed not to contact him.". I also hadn't given permission for them to reference me in their report in any way. Dan fumbled through a meek response that the investigators thought it would be a good idea. I snapped, "You can justify all kinds of things that other people tell you to do. I told you I did not want my elderly, estranged father contacted, and you agreed. That's institutional abuse".

Libby, as always, listened in. It was like a rerun of this terrible show we kept playing over and over again. Dan Scheibe would do something he knew was wrong, following through on what Paul or Bruce or now investigators told him to do, and Libby got to listen in and hear me blow up at them.

Of course, Dan Scheibe had reason to believe that my parents, and my father, in particular, would go along with their efforts to make this all look small. School administrators had been successful in securing his compliance in the 1990s. I'd told Dan Scheibe and Paul Lannon, at the onset of our direct communications, that I did not want my parents involved. They agreed to not disturb them. My parents had proven so unhelpful to me at the time. I knew they carried some weird mix of guilt, defensiveness, and avoidance that would only confuse my efforts now.

I was carrying on as an adult to create a new conclusion, despite their lack of support.

Remember, Dan Scheibe had given assurances for my safety when we first spoke in early 2018. Yet, he'd been party to all kinds of moral and legal wrongs since. "*So and so told me to do it*" is never an acceptable excuse from a child who has done wrong. It is even less acceptable from an adult, especially one acting as the leader of a school.

Since we'd come this far, in his delivering bad news, I asked Dan to tell me the statement. It was something to the effect of 'we wouldn't do anything to hurt Vanessa...' which morphed into "We wouldn't have done anything Vanessa didn't want us to do". Of course, they all had. They had done two things I didn't want them to do: taking me away from my friends and education - and keeping a child molester on campus despite my pleading. If they were trying to ease their own guilty conscience publicly now, they sure as Fuck were not going to do it at my expense.

~ ~ ~

Dan was stuck, caught in yet another moral and ethical violation. I said firmly and abruptly, "If you print any statement that even subtly implies that leaving was my idea, I will file a law suit for defamation and other charges" I enjoyed a moment's pause and declared, "I have to go.". I hung up the phone.

I called Noah and left him a message. Then, I called the other lawyers I had on hand in Boston. I said the school was releasing their report the next day, and it could contain specific defamation. I wanted us to be ready. I went ahead and left my dad a few messages, too. I hadn't called my father by my own urges in well over a decade. I said to his voicemail, "I don't know what you're doing, but you need to call them right now and tell them they are not allowed to print that comment. I am ready to sue anyone who tries to protect their reputation at my expense at this point. Including you".

That night, the lawyers, my supporters, and I all went to sleep awaiting the school's next move. Lawrence Academy officials were threatening to harm me and preparing to make themselves look as good as possibly publicly. All in one evening.

To be thorough, I woke early and sent one more message by email to Dan Scheibe, Paul Lannon, Bruce MacNeil, and Libby Margraf by the start of the east coast workday:

Thu, Apr 25, 2019, 6:04 AM

Let me be very clear.

If you publish a statement that even subtly suggests it was my decision to leave Lawrence Academy after the abuse of 1993-94, I will file a lawsuit for defamation. I will include charges for negligence, breach of confidentiality, slander and more.

I have been high-minded and kind. I have a large and loyal following in The Amends Project.

You would be wise to weigh your options carefully.

~ ~ ~

A new Lowell Sun reporter named Jon Winkler called me, as well. With Rick Sobey now at The Boston Herald, The Sun needed someone else to carry on with the series. I was hiking with our dog on nearby Galbraith Mountain when he called and asked me for a statement. Early on, I'd reached out to over a dozen reporters to pay attention to this story. By now, new, unknown reporters were coming to me.

I answered his questions and stayed focused on the more pressing issue: the failure of response. I told Jon Winkler I'd founded a nonprofit called The Amends Project to address the cover-up problem and was working on an initiative called The Justice CORPS. I said I too would be releasing a tally of all the numbers I'd gathered on the incidents at the school. I told him people had been contacting me for months to share stories. He asked, "Where will you be releasing that?". I said, "On The Amends Project website."

~ ~ ~

Even with all the communication with the school leading up to the report's release, I still had to ask a friend to forward me their statement and link to their report. No one from Lawrence Academy sent it to me. Clearly, it wasn't me they were apologizing to. My biggest priority was learning whether they had taken the extra liberty to print that misleading statement. Was I going to have to sue them? Were they really going to try to make me look like a liar to support their "disagreement" defense? How much bang were they trying to get for their "we own this story" buck?

I scanned the report, which contained nothing new or surprising to me, looking frantically for the defaming statement. It was not there. I was immensely relieved.

It turns out, they absolutely *could* edit the contents of that report if it served them. The call from Dan Scheibe had been risk-assessment. They tested the waters, for how I would respond - and I said I would sue. So, they decided they'd better not take the risk. This was every bit the proof I needed to confirm that they controlled the content, the timing, the outcome of this report.

Noah, I could tell, was crushed. He'd allowed himself to hope for the goodness in my approach to be reflected back by a school he had loved. He saw me taking a higher road, and he longed to see them step up onto it with me. They had done the opposite. He never told me directly, but I believe Noah lost the last threads of faith in the school that day.

~ ~ ~

The report tallied four accounts of abuse by Pete Regis from former students (Sybil and I, the woman who'd thanked me, and another classmate at the time not included). It gave a notable amount of space to describing Pete's shop - far more attention than it gave to Steve Hahn or what he knew or did. It included a statement, "students were made aware [of Pete's behavior] at an assembly or in advising" Who had made them aware? Not school leaders. I had made them aware. That would be confusing and misleading to readers.

Student A submitted this, "There was a backlash against the students who made the allegations, and the school did not address this."

Best of all was watching the number of visitors to The Amends Project page rise and rise and rise. Every time I checked the stats, the bar had jumped another inch. It reached an all-time high that day. If Lawrence Academy said, "This is what happened," hundreds of people then wanted to know, "What does Vanessa say?"

Here is what I said:

Week 51: By the Numbers

"He who goes looking for a lack of evidence will surely find it."

"He who writes the check shall be exonerated."

7

7: number of times former student Vanessa Osage approached Lawrence Academy headmaster Steven Hahn in his office, from 1994-2000, pleading first for her protection, and then, for the protection of incoming students.

7

7: number of years Lawrence Academy officials decided to knowingly employ a documented child molester on campus.

300

300: number, as an estimate, of students, faculty & staff in attendance in the Lawrence Academy auditorium, on December 10, 2001, in which former student Vanessa Osage (then, 23) gave a speech revealing that leadership had been knowingly exposing them to the dangers of a child molester on campus.

(Peter Regis was finally let go, only when she was on her way to campus from California and could not be reached; he was dismissed on "permanent, long-term disability")

4

4: number of sexual misconduct incidents, by former employee Peter Regis, recorded by Sanghavi Law Office during their investigation.

9

9: number of of sexual misconduct incidents, by former employee Peter Regis, tallied by alumni in the fall of 2018 (individual accounts by different people)

5+

5+: number of alumni who refused to participate in that investigation/internal report on a matter of principle.

1

1: number in rank that "lack of trust" was cited as a reason to not participate.

19

19: number of alumni who have pledged, in writing, to not donate to Lawrence Academy again, or until they make this situation right.

11

11: number of people who have contacted me, Vanessa Osage, privately since the Lowell Sun feature article of May 27, 2018 to concur and share their **stories of painful cover-up behavior by Lawrence Academy** (both former and current administrations)

2017

2017: year of most recent account, given by the parent of a former student by phone, about current Lawrence Academy leadership's efforts to silence, bully, "buy them out" with a tuition refund, and more, following an assault on their child by a faculty member.

1991, 1993, 1994, 1995, 2014, 2015, 2016

: years that represent the remaining cover-up stories shared about Lawrence Academy

3

3: number of stories shared, **with accounts from 2014-2017**, of Lawrence Academy officials offering families free or reimbursed tuition in exchange for silence (leaving and/or not pressing charges) for child abuse on campus.

22+

22+: number of hours I, Vanessa Osage, have spent on the phone since May 2018, with alumni, former Trustees and/or parents of recent Lawrence Academy students; to console, affirm and corroborate their stories of unethical behavior by administration following abuse of themselves or their child.

(number does not include hours spent in collaboration with other alumni, professionals, and child safety advocates from around the country, to address this)

Unknown

:number of ways, or extent to which, Dan Scheibe, Paul Lannon and/or Bruce MacNeil will attempt to defame or discredit former Lawrence Academy student, Vanessa Osage, '96.

Unknown

:extended costs of current leadership choosing to mislead, hide facts, silence, avoid, bully and/or coerce *any member of the Lawrence Academy community.*

Unknown

:the quantitative impact on families, who must question whether to believe a former student (students) or Lawrence Academy school leaders who are responsible for the care of their kids.

2

2: number of years since headmaster Dan Scheibe asked people to come forward.

2

2: number of private, independent high schools from across the nation, to be engaged in the pilot program of The Justice CORPS – the Committee to Oversee the Rights & Protections of Students, for the 2019-2020 school year.

4

4: number of times The Justice CORPS model was proposed to Lawrence Academy, as part of resolution, from July 2018 – February 2019; also the number of times rejected.

3

3: the current number of professional Advisors to the nonprofit, The Amends Project, in addition to myself, who are lending their time and expertise to seeing that positive change is secured at private, independent high schools, for the sake of kids and families.
(number does not include additional people who offer their high quality support, expertise and wise counsel, behind the scenes)

0

0: Zero, the cost of looking at what people do, instead of what they say, to inform your decisions about what is true.

1

1: the number of readers it takes to make a significant, positive impact on the outcomes at Lawrence Academy (and beyond).

You Are 1

Stay tuned, dear reader . . .

Then, I found Jon Winkler's article in The Lowell Sun.

Please note, as he introduces me, he (or new Editor Tom Zuppa) chooses to take out all information about The Amends Project nonprofit, The Justice CORPS Initiative and my report on the website. He, or they, chose the dismissively simple word, victim.

NEWS I LOCAL NEWS

Report: Lawrence Academy worker exposed himself to students in 1990s[18]

...Vanessa Osage, one of the two victims who came forward with allegations when she was a student in the 1990s, said on Thursday that she was aware of the investigation but chose not to participate on the principle that she believed the investigation was a "diversion" from where focus needed to be.

She told her story to The Sun in May 2018, with another victim coming forward with allegations against Regis two months later.

[18] Jon Winkler, The Lowell Sun, April 26, 2018, https://theamendsproject.com/press/

Osage told The Sun last year that she was seeking a $500,000 settlement from the school for losses and damages. She said on Thursday that she still expects the school to settle with her [*"because it's the right thing to do" was my complete sentence*] and that the monetary amount of the settlement has been lowered to "20 percent of the original demand."

"The more important investigation is to the extent of which current and former headmasters mistreated students and families to cover up instances of abuse," Osage said. "This investigation only arose in response to another alumna coming forward."

Osage had been trying to convince Hahn to address the allegations since June 1997 [*actually, starting in May 1994*] and even told an auditorium full of students at the school her story in December 2001.

"They seem to take credit for the speech that I gave in 2001 at an assembly at age 23 after seven years of expecting them to do the right thing," Osage added, referring to the school. "There needs to be a more thorough look at the failures of responding."

I asked Bruce McNeil again that they settle with me following the investigation. The report had confirmed four separate accounts as "credible", nearly halfway to the nine I'd confirmed in conversations with alumni. Bruce MacNeil kept me waiting, and then sent me lengthy emails recapping their main points:

1. They still believed their "full and final settlement" of $75,000 was fair
2. That he believed they had acknowledged my efforts and apologized to me
3. They would be making no further public statements

I honestly feel that same old fear now as I write. Were Dan Scheibe and Bruce MacNeil actually starting to believe the lies they told themselves and the school community?

Truly, it upsets the natural order in the universe to mess with truth in this way. How had they not yet learned?

Wed, May 15, 2019, 11:13 AM

to Bruce, Dan, Paul

Gentlemen,

Common sense tells me that if you had intended to apologize to me at all, you would have included me in the email to the community.

I disagree with your assessment of the situation entirely.

You have not acknowledged the backlash or my efforts.

Given this, I will move forward accordingly.

Thank you,

Vanessa

Would Never = Hasn't Yet

"I can't believe that!" said Alice.
"Can't you?" the Queen said in a pitying tone.
"Try again: draw a long breath, and shut your eyes."
Alice laughed. "There's no use trying," she said:
"one *can't* believe impossible things."

"I daresay you haven't had much practice,"
said the Queen.
"When I was your age, I always did it
for half-an-hour a day.
Why, sometimes I've believed as many as
six impossible things before breakfast."

– Lewis Carrol, *Through the Looking Glass*

Many people had suggested I connect with the leader of a child safety organization in New England. "Oh, you should talk to so-and-so" was often the beginning of great collaborations and joint efforts. So, of course, I followed through. She'd had great success in training staff at schools on sexual abuse and appropriate response. Her assessments had shown that understanding of what to do increased dramatically following the training. We emailed for a time, and at last, we were talking by phone.

She and I were in conversation for over an hour, in what became (to my surprise) something of a debate. Without expecting it, we learned we had fundamentally different approaches to effecting positive change in schools. She worked within structures as they were. I was advocating for a root-level (radical, by definition) overhaul in how we delegate decision-making power.

Both were important. We just marveled at the polarity of our entry-points. Two of her comments have stayed with me. One: "Schools would never allow someone outside of them decide how to respond to abuse," and later, as a lovely counterpart, "Maybe what you're suggesting is so ahead of your time, I just can't grasp it yet."

That kind of comment, for me, is a testimony to humility and personal security that I find awe-inspiring.

"I don't get you, but maybe it's because you are seeing further than I am currently seeing." Wow.

It was a great experience of seeing that, while we can disagree fundamentally, there is always a way to come around to mutual respect. I trust that she and I will meet again on the road to positive reform. She fully earned my respect that day.

~ ~ ~

I mused on The Amends Project website:

I've been thinking a lot about the statement, "That would never happen."

Indeed, we do count on those who see beyond a current situation to what could be and what needs to happen. It wasn't all that long ago when people were reconciling these shifts:

"Women would never own property." became "a woman hasn't owned property yet." **Then, she had.**

An African-American man would never be president" became "an African-American man hasn't been president yet. **Then, he had.**

And on it goes. It's important to remember this long-range view, as we move forward...

"Private schools would never choose to be transparent about abuses and how they respond to them." has become, "a private school hasn't accepted transparency yet."

Until then, two had.

If we only look backward to inform what is possible, we miss so many opportunities for accelerating progress now.

Stories We Tell - Misleading Public Statements

When we accept vague or hollow language from people in power, we collectively lower our standards as a society.

From the Justice CORPS article of April 2, 2019:

In a statement last year to The Sun, Lawrence Academy Head of School Dan Scheibe wrote, "Had the same set of circumstances presented themselves today, there is no question that *we would have* immediately terminated the staff member from employment at the school."

Which, of course, begs the question: what if it was your nephew?

Hypothetical statements are unverifiable, which makes them hollow and useless to anyone but the speaker. Any public declaration that uses the word *would* is an attempt to capture future credit for a present-tense unknown. This is the flip-side of *would never*. It all speaks to possibility. Yet, in this way, it can also thwart progress.

You just don't know what you would do until you do it. I remember an elementary school teacher posing a "*What would you do?*' question to the class, where we each had the opportunity to answer in front of everyone. It was an imagined test of character and strength. It was hypothetical.

I recall listening to my classmates declare and even boast of the courage they would demonstrate. I knew instantly I was not hopping in on this one, so I listened and observed. As each spoke, my internal judgment or reality-check brought me back continuously to one thought, 'You don't know *what* you would do.' Those words-spoken were intentions or expressions of aspirational values at best. For that moment, it was a chance to possibly claim credit publicly for a heroic deed not yet done.

Author Tommy Baker spoke with entrepreneurial podcast host Matt Gottesman in 2019, urging aspiring business-owners to not say what they are going to do online before they do it. Making those statement actually led to lowered success rates. He says, "There is danger in declaration." He clarifies that the power in declaring lies only in speaking it to the people who will hold you accountable.

When leaders of elite schools make unverified public declarations, so far, it has been with the confidence that they will not be held accountable.

Baker illustrates, "People go on Facebook [and say], 'I'm gonna run a 20-mile marathon; I'm gonna launch a six/seven-figure business'. You look at the comments - this person hasn't done one thing - what are the comments saying? 'Matt, you're so disciplined. Matt, you're so committed. Matt, that's amazing.'

"So, they're getting acknowledgment for a future result they actually haven't created.", Baker continues. "The research is really clear about that: it actually demotivates them because they feel like they already got the benefit."

"There's a neurological connection," Gottesman adds, "with saying it, is giving them an endorphin rush of doing it. So it's actually a false sense of success or accomplishment. Well, therefore, subconsciously, they don't even have to do it. They don't even realize, since it's happening on a subconscious level."

Let's realize what is happening. Hypothetical *would* statements from those in power bring us down as a nation. The only way these words can lift us is when they line up with action. Consider, if we let these public statements be *The Stories We Tell* now, what will the shape of our world be two hundred years from today?

Intersections - Internal Biases, External Consequences

"Justice will not be served until
those who are unaffected are as outraged
as those who are."

— Benjamin Franklin

Oh, and when I returned home to Washington, after that Open House trip in the fall, I walked down to my local police station and filed a report of "Bullying" by Lawrence Academy of Groton, Massachusetts.

I knew how to do that now. During my brief time working with Mitchell Garabedian, I'd learned that you need a police report in order to file a lawsuit in these cases. It was a formality. I was 40 years old when I learned this - and in no universe of awareness would I have ever known it at 14, 15, or 16. This is one gap The Justice CORPS fills: informing young people of their rights and the legal process of reporting abuse. So, I walked into a Washington state police station in 2017 and filed that report on Pete Regis.

Making that first report was downright awkward. Many times, I had to explain to the officer that I was doing this as part of a lawsuit against a school. Yes, a school in Massachusetts. Yes, for incidents in 1993-94. After

Lawrence Academy decision-makers messed with me in the fall of 2018, though, I was easy and confident walking into the local police station again.

Of course, I can do this - knowingly utilizing the system to my potential benefit - because I am perceived as white. I am of a racial group that can rely on these assumptions of safety. That is not the case for everyone. People of color in this country have come to rightly fear our "justice" system as much as any unknown predator or violent criminal. Their very lives have been at stake.

In 2018, child abuse in the United States disproportionately affected Native and Black youth at nearly twice the rate of white children (15.2% Native, 14% African American vs. 8.2% white)[19]. LGBTQ people also suffer far higher rates of abuse and discrimination. Justice is not yet equally distributed.

~ ~ ~

In early 2020, I attended a training on The Groundwater Approach to understanding racial inequities presented by the Racial Equity Institute at the community college in Bellingham, WA. When something goes wrong, their metaphor suggests, it's not about the individual fish; it's something in the groundwater. They defined Institutional Oppression as collective group prejudice that is backed by legal authority and institutional control.

When an institution structures its decision-making behind the secrecy shield of "handling it internally", schools run the risk of allowing racial biases to play out in the lives of young people with real, detrimental results.

My insight into the intersection of race and institutional control comes from both heard and lived experience. Alumni of Lawrence Academy tell of the African-American male student who was "made an example" in the 90s after an assault allegation, "and immediately expelled. In the same year,

[19] Statista, January 16, 2020, https://www.statista.com/statistics/254857/child-abuse-rate-in-the-us-by-race-ethnicity/

the storyteller alleges, a white male student with family and money connections was "covered for" and, most tragically, emboldened to abuse repeatedly at Lawrence Academy.

Internal biases had very real external consequences for students and the school community.

When I sat as a registered guest at Open House in the auditorium in 2018, I watched a female, African-American student in a panel of six young people on stage. She said that Lawrence Academy gave her the feeling she could use her voice to make positive change in the world. The moderator swooned. Then, less than an hour later, Lawrence Academy officials sent police to arrest me on the school lawn for speaking of the positive change I was advocating on campus.

The Racial Equity Institute poses a follow-up question, regarding their definition of Institutional Oppression: *Who was it set up to advantage?*

The question I offer, as creator and facilitator of The Justice CORPS Initiative is this: How could the very person a system is structured to advantage be the best one to decide how abuse is handled on campus?

They can't.

Students and families need somewhere else to go. They need a system that neutralizes for the effects of systemic racism, elitism, and sexism. As we begin to understand the danger of these biases, our new systems can reflect a commitment to justice in every choice.

This is where we now must go.

Who Can We Tell?

"Did you tell anyone?", asks Boston Globe reporter
Sacha Pfieffer, of a man who had endured abuse by a priest.
He replies, *"Like who, a priest?"*

"Who was I going to tell, the invisible DA?",
asks a Hollywood actress, rhetorically,
about her options for reporting abuse
by Harvey Weinstein.

"I don't know who to tell, or what to do",
said Chessy Prout, in her book,
"I Have the Right To", about
sexual assault at St. Paul's School.

In all the stories I've come across about sexual assault, harassment, or abuse in an institutional setting, this same question surfaces over and over again. I know, some of you must be thinking, 'the police!'. It simply doesn't happen that way. I have to say, it doesn't happen for good reason. Even beyond the tragic police brutality against minority racial groups, there is a broader reason for young people.

The 2016 Boston Globe report on retaliation comments on the not-reporting phenomenon, "This pattern of reticence is consistent with a 2004 national study that found only 6 to 10 percent of students abused by educators report it to someone who can do something about it."

Why?

Power imbalances. When an adult has overpowered a young person, it then becomes very unlikely that the young person will seek out someone in a position of power to help them. It's the dynamic that was abused. So, instinctively, we conclude that the same dynamic would not suddenly heal.

The Providence (Rhode Island) Journal reported on incidents at St. George's School[20], "The abuse they experienced involved not only physical acts of sexual assault (as horrible as those were), but something that, for many, was even worse: betrayal at the hands of an adult entrusted with their care, at a school where they saw few, if any places to turn for help."

People just don't know where to go. Imagine a student tells a school staff member who is more accessible than a higher-up administrator. That employee will likely still face a series of internal pressures to keep quiet or 'let them take it from there'. So many people at Lawrence Academy who'd heard about Sybil and me confronting Pete Regis in 1994 reflexively believed "they would handle it". Handling it, of course, becomes too open to interpretation - too subject to internal biases. Like the policy states, "the school determines whether to investigate".

Neither Sybil nor I chose to "bring our concerns to an adult" as one community message from Dan Scheibe wrongly stated. Our friend heard about us confronting Pete Regis. She told a teacher, and the news eventually reached headmaster Steve Hahn. Then, they tricked us into the surprise meeting, with zero follow up on what happens next. All the while, Pete Regis roamed the campus free from consequence.

In an article on the Spotlight film,[21] *The Guardian* reporter Henry Barnes writes of movie co-writer Josh Singer's motivation to tell this story, "It

---

[20] Karen Lee Ziner, The Providence Journal, September 1, 2016, https://www.providencejournal.com/news/20160901/st-georges-sex-abuse-scandal-report-excoriates-school-for-decades-of-unchecked-abuse

[21] Henry Barnes, The Guardian, January 13, 2016, https://www.theguardian.com/film/2016/jan/13/spotlight-reporters-uncovered-catholic-child-abuse-boston-globe

was this implicit deference by the police, attorneys and, to some degree, the press that interested Singer in the story. In a key scene, a lawyer who represents the victims says: "It takes a village to raise a child. It takes a village to abuse one."

"That collective looking away was always interesting," Singer says.

~ ~ ~

What does implicit deference look like? Police approaching me on the Lawrence Academy campus at Open House, after receiving an order to wrongfully arrest. These officers likely knew there was no cause for arrest, yet deferred to school officials, beyond their code of duty. What is collective looking away? You might have your own painful example. It's the moment when a bystander remains silent because s/he is receiving a signal that abuse is tolerated. So, what can we do?

We empower people with alternatives to safely, honestly handle it together.

From the short film on Restorative Justice by Brave New Films[22], the narrator begins, "More than half of victims of violent crime don't even call the police in the first place (citing 52% of all crime in the US as going unreported). They prefer *nothing* to everything we have to offer."

"The vast majority of crime survivors' pain goes unhealed. What the existence of Restorative Justice means is that we can no longer pretend we don't know what to do."

The same can now be said about The Justice CORPS model. This is something else we can do.

~ ~ ~

---

[22] Brave New Films, September 13, 2016, https://www.youtube.com/watch?v=8N3LihLvfao

So, imagine a diverse group of adults and college-aged interns exists solely for protecting your rights as a teenager. No getting in trouble if drugs or alcohol were involved. No threats to keep you off the team or give you a bad grade, or remove your financial aid if you speak up. You are a child or an adolescent, and someone put you in a vulnerable position. You felt scared and powerless, and something terrible happened.

Now, you have options. You learned your rights in assembly and how the process looks from this group of volunteers from an outside organization. They all feel more like social-workers or counselors than police. Blaming you is not even an option. They're not even part of the school.

They know all about these things and will calmly record the information and explain your options to you. You'll understand the process from there. You also know in advance that school leaders will be graded on how well they respond. Everyone needs to live up to a high standard. That information, once it reaches decision-makers, is free from gender, racial, sexual-orientation or socioeconomic bias. It will have your age only.

Of course, at the bottom of every failure to respond well is the ability for leaders to ask, *"Who was it?"* and craft their response accordingly. This is where the net of justice falls out from under us, as a society today. There is no room for abuse of power to say, *"It depends who it is"*. That's the dark side of "handling it internally": room for biases to inform how justice is or is not served. That is the old practice, now falling away.

In The Justice CORPS model, schools start the year with a high score of 10. Then, for every incident of abuse, a deduction of 1-3 points is recorded. Every incident of abuse carries the same weight, regardless of who enacted it and who suffered. Consider that again: every incident carries the same weight. That is the kind of logic that keeps kids feeling upright in this world.

The "who" is kept of out records for just this reason. For example, data of a report to the Justice CORPS would read:

Student, age 15, made a complaint about inappropriate touching by a teacher in a locker room at the campus sports complex on 5/13

Report received to Justice CORPS on 5/22.

Student chose to involve their parents. Family is undecided about pressing charges.

Incident Point Deduction: - 3

Student, age 13, made a report of sexual coercion (2nd degree) by a student, age 18, during a school outing on 4/4-4/5.

Report received to Justice CORPS on 4/8.

Student has not chosen to involve parents.

Incident Point Deduction: - 2

Students (not school officials) choose whether or not to involve parents because the students' rights have priority. If drugs or alcohol were involved, a young person can still feel safe in reporting, without fear of consequence for other offenses. The dignity or a young person and the sovereignty of a family are both preserved by leaving that choice where it belongs.

A trained investigator serves on The Justice CORPS team, yet remains unknown to school officials. This person can do their job without pressure to arrive at a particular conclusion. There is no reason for school officials to be involved in an investigation. A vested interest can only interfere. So, the real work of justice happens outside the influence of affluence.

Control can feel like security until the urge to control gets out of control. At that point, we have to step in as people around an issue and redistribute power.

A tally of incidents is sent to school leaders monthly. Then, their response either meets, exceeds, or falls short of the Recommendations laid out by the Independent Schools Task Force of 2018. A system of Recovery

Points allows schools to shine in what they really can control: how well they respond.

Meeting these guidelines can earn schools back 1-3 points, canceling out the negative numbers and the negative effects on the community. Meeting guidelines minimally earns one point. Meeting them thoroughly earns two. Utilizing Restorative Justice earns schools three Recovery Points.

A subsequent report might read:

Student, age 15, made a complaint about inappropriate touching by a teacher in a locker room at the campus sports complex on 5/13

Report received to Justice CORPS on 5/22.

Student chose to involve their parents. Family is undecided about pressing charges.

Incident Point Deduction: - 3

Recovery Point Earned: + 3

Net impact score: 0

Student, age 13, made a report of sexual coercion (2nd degree) by a student, age 18, during a school outing on 4/4-4/5.

Report received to Justice CORPS on 4/8.

Student has not chosen to involve parents.

Incident Point Deduction: - 2

Recovery Point Earned: 1

Net Impact Score: -1

Restorative Justice not only heals communities in the wake of abuse, it allows young people to keep a nuanced view of themselves as they grow into adulthood. One unfortunate encounter can leave someone a victim and someone a perpetrator in the current system. Yet, through Restorative Justice, young people can find the necessary compassion for themselves and another, and grow as whole humans - learning from mistakes, with support.

An attorney in the field also assured me, The Justice CORPS system can work just as well for student-to-student incidents as staff-to-student. In the latter, Restorative Justice can also mean an adult who is ill with behavioral disease can better seek treatment, and stop themselves from harming again. Even employed adults can get out of control and need real scaffolding to stop abusive behaviors.

Mandated Reporter Status remains active for all adults in the employed care and education of children. The Justice CORPS simply means a greater number of kids won't fall through the old cracks in the existing system.

In 2018, I also collaborated with a local filmmaker friend to prepare to offer (the first two) participating schools a short promotional documentary film to highlight their experience of embracing transparency in response. I am so eager to bring a positive exposure campaign to this issue around the country.

Please visit https://theamendsproject.com/justice-corps/ to see the latest version of The Justice CORPS Initiative proposal.

~ ~ ~

Now, imagine again that you are a young person at a private high school and someone put you in a vulnerable position. Your school is enrolled in an oversight and transparency system called The Justice CORPS.

You have somewhere to go.

You saw this group on stage and when you go online to make a report, you choose which person you feel safest with from a drop-down menu. You have guarantees that this information will not be lost. You have caring, impartial people to guide you through. Your school will be graded on how well they do.

Everyone is expected to live up to a high standard, including school leaders.

Imagine how safe you could truly feel on campus. No matter who you are. The score for incidents is the same, regardless of race, gender, sexual orientation, religious or political affiliation, socio-economic status or even academic standing. When it comes to Justice, violations against any young person all carry the exact same weight in a true community. No matter who you love, what racial heritage you claim, how much your parents make or who they know: True safeguards for Justice.

Justice CORPS Video

"If we make power invisible, racism thrives"

— A Nation at Risk: The Imperative for Educational Reform, 1983

"We can only solve the problem that we truly see."

A friend made a wonderful suggestion on a hike one day. She reflected, "You need a more digestible way for people to understand your vision. You can see it, but others can't grasp it completely. What about one of those white board animation videos?" She was right, and I loved it. The idea brought me back to the very early stages of seeking alternate resolution - when I imagined going public with a simple, light-hearted video. I wanted something that tells a hard story in a simple, easy medium.

So, I withdrew money from the GoFundMe donation account and hired a freelance animator/videographer on Fiverr (for $65). She lived in Saudi Arabia, with a precisely twelve hour time difference to Pacific Standard Time in Washington, USA. Working together proved challenging in only that way. Despite different primary languages, she created a beautiful work of whiteboard animation to teach and describe the solution I'd created. People were not going to sit down and read a 10-page pdf - but they would watch a cute, 4-minute video.

I wrote a script, and imagined all the accompanying visuals. It would outline the problem, and more importantly, the solution.

I chose a male narrator, which evoked a range of opinions in those close to me. Most wanted to hear my voice. Some understood the goals behind the choice, and called it "effective". As Jackson Katz of MVP Strategies says, in the privileged group, for men, the word "gender" means women. That way, men can conclude that "gender violence issues" don't apply to them. I knew all too well how this problem could be overlooked as an issue not relevant to (certain) men. Again, one in six boys are sexually abused before their 18th birthday.

This solution had to speak to those who were able to make the choice to implement it. Men still held the majority of decision-making power in these institutions. I saw first-hand how some females had deferred to the men, at great expense to children.

This was about and highly relevant to men. So, they needed to be able to hear it. The narrator reads:

"What is The Justice CORPS?

A solution. The answer to a decades-long problem. It's the moral of the story...

Say something bad happens at a school. A kid goes to what he considers the responsible adult. Then, there is a Conflict.

This adult thinks of the kid, yes. He also thinks of his job, the school's reputation, and the endowment. Let's assume, for a moment, he is torn. He might tell the child "It wasn't a big deal" or "I'm sure they didn't mean it." This adult might offer the child's family some money under the table... "Shh, that should keep this quiet now."

Then what?

That child loses faith in adults and society. He and his family lose trust in the school. "We are so grand!" Discord grows as people recognize the painful contrast between word and action.

Then! The child may grow up having normalized corruption and secrecy. If he makes a mistake in his job - he will draw on his education to inform his decisions."Oh, let's just store those files in the shredder room."

Institutions crumble, and societies weaken - unless we turn this all around now.

The Justice CORPS is a transparency and oversight model that opens up channels of healthy, fresh air alongside these institutions.

Non-affiliated adults volunteer to receive and track reports of abuse. Then, they record whether schools fall short, meet or exceed guidelines laid out by the Independent Schools Task Force of 2018. But first, the school year starts with an all-school assembly where kids learn their rights, meet Justice CORPS members, learn how to report incidents and understand what happens once the process begins. A second assembly is held mid-year to review.

The Justice CORPS is the Committee to Oversee the Rights & Protections of Students - and they serve both schools and families.

When a school participates in the Justice CORPS model, they take a brave step to say, "We care so sincerely about the wellbeing of our students that we want to demonstrate honor on all levels." That makes schools stronger - and more attractive to prospective families.

Schools can exceed the guidelines by utilizing Restorative Justice. A modern version of an ancient model for repair and peacemaking, Restorative Justice responsibly addresses the harms caused and brings in the larger community to achieve true resolution. Restorative Justice practices can reduce recidivism by 83%, and has a 98% satisfaction rate among participants who were harmed.

The Justice CORPS model is a three year commitment. Why three years? Experts understand that once kids are empowered to speak up about abuse, reporting will rise. "Wait, we can talk about this?!" So, three year cycles give enough time for numbers to stabilize while abuse is prevented.

Best of all! Those schools that can reduce the true incidence of abuse by 50% or more in three year cycles earn a Seal of Excellence in Child Safety from a supporting organization. We can only solve the problem that we truly see.

The Justice CORPS, an initiative of the nonprofit The Amends Project, offers a solution and way through to renewed strength on the other side.

visit www.theamendsproject.com to apply for participation in the pilot program.

To give to this vision, visit Support the Movement on The Amends Project website.

~ ~ ~

I emailed a link for the video to everyone at Lawrence Academy. I'd pieced together now that my Amends Project email had been blocked by school leaders. I'm almost embarrassed to admit I'd missed just how "insecure" those work emails would be. If I contacted existing faculty to solicit their support, they would have to self-censor their response - out of fear of retaliation for fraternizing with the enemy. It didn't occur to me that Dan Scheibe, or others, would retain the ability to read people's emails or to block senders.

These moments started to echo of cruel dictatorships I'd learned about in history. I didn't want to consider or believe this. Yet, it was real. It was, after all, written right into the Declaration of Independence:

> *We have Petitioned for Redress in the most humble terms: Our repeated Petitions have been answered only by repeated injury. A Prince whose character is thus marked by every act which may define a Tyrant, is unfit to be the ruler of a free people.*

Once I understood this, I bypassed the block by sending The Justice CORPS video link through a new email address.

I had to confirm with a former teacher, a current staff member who I count as an ally, by phone to learn whether it had come through. Finally, it had.

~ ~ ~

One day soon after, I sat in my car by a newly opened bayside park in my hometown of Bellingham, WA. I'd driven down there for a brief rest between seeing clients and teaching. In the quiet calm of my lunch break in the car, the urge came so suddenly: I wanted to talk to Jamie Baker, the Assistant Headmaster I'd met at Lawrence Academy's Open House.

To my surprise, she picked up. Again, sadly, I understood now that people in the school were afraid to talk to me. They feared - unfortunately, for good reason - suffering repercussions for doing so. If the school wouldn't apologize for retaliation, they were essentially saying they believed their retaliations were warranted.

Jamie answered.

I was so happy to talk to her. She was hushed in her voice initially, almost hurrying through the willingness to connect. But, she admitted she wanted to talk because she'd seen the video. She was all encouragement, "The tone is just right" and "it gets the message across in a way that really allows people to hear it".

She said I needed to just get that video in front of as many people as possible. She encouraged me to post it on YouTube. I told her I was trying to raise $250,000 to fund a pilot of the program for three years. She asked if I could propose the school fund The Justice CORPS as resolution. I told her I had asked, and they had declined. She mused with both disappointment and an undertone of hope, "It would be such an elegant conclusion."

Jamie's heartfelt clarity snapped me out of the pain of the present moment. All of Lawrence Academy officials' cruel, unethical moves to get me to go away suddenly receded as my vision refocused. She helped to reorient me to my long-term goals. Staying focused while an institution bullies you takes a vast reserve of energy. Jamie's calm voice and clear-sighted support refilled those reserves for me that day.

On Apology

"The non-apologizer walks
on a tight rope of defensiveness,
above a huge canyon of low self-esteem."

— Harriet Lerner

"What doesn't bend, breaks. What doesn't bend breaks."

— Ani DiFranco

The very same month, in May of 2019, *This American Life* aired a new episode called, *"Get a Spine!"* with the story of the genuine public apology in Act One, *Finally*.

It involved a writer named Meghan Ganz, currently Executive Producer on *It's Always Sunny in Philadelphia* - and her former boss: writer, actor, co-creator and showrunner for the NBC show, "Community", Dan Harmon. He had many writers working with him on the show, but he was essentially the boss. The incidents had happened years earlier, and their road to the sincere apology was long and uncertain, not unlike mine with Lawrence Academy.

Nancy Updike tells the story. She says, "I listened in headphones on the subway [to Dan Harmon's public apology on his podcast *Harmon Town* in 2018], and it was the auditory equivalent of seeing a snow leopard stroll through the subway car."

"It was not curt or vague. It was not a lawyered up mess of non-contrition in the passive voice.

From a public statement written by Paul Lannon, attorney for Lawrence Academy: *"The school did not do enough to prevent such harm and to protect the students in its care, and we apologize for those failures."*

"It was a true reckoning. Publicly and fully accepted by the person who had been wronged. She forgave him. That almost never happens - a public apology that lands.

\- - -

Harmon says, "I was attracted to an employee... The most clinical way I can put it is, I was attracted to a writer that I had power over because I was a showrunner. And I knew enough to know that these feelings were bad news - and so I did the cowardly, easiest, laziest thing you could do with feelings like that and I didn't deal with them. And in not dealing with them, I made everybody else deal with them. Especially her."

His live-in girlfriend at the time asked if he had feelings for that young writer he was always talking about. He admits in this apology that he lied to her by saying No. "Because the trick is - if you lie to yourself, you can lie to everybody else - it's really easy.", he says.

"So, that's what I continued to do. Telling myself - and anybody that threatened to confront me with it - that if you thought what I was doing was creepy or flirty or unprofessional, then it's because you were the sexist. You were jealous; I'm a mentor; I'm a feminist. It's your problem, not mine. You're the one that actually is seeing things through that lens. And so, I let myself keep doing it.", Harmon says.

Here, Dan Harmon is acknowledging a few of those D-word tactics also used often by Lawrence Academy officials: diversion, discrediting, and, most of all, denial.

As I listened, I noticed the balance in his approach. On one end of not apologizing is an arrogant denial - on the other is self-effacing groveling. Both extremes avoid the real work of staying present to what happened and the struggle to own it maturely. The latter can seem humble, yet is often a tool to evoke sympathy from the listener, ultimately avoiding responsibility again. Dan Harmon doesn't do this. He finds that middle ground and speaks from there.

Continuing with his accounting of the incidents, he refers to the very clear and repeated ways this employee told him that any preferential treatment would be damaging to her as a writer. She was articulate, forthright, and insistent. Harmon says:

"I just didn't hear it. And it's because it didn't profit me to hear it - and this was, after all, happening to me, right?"

He clings to this pursuit of his employee, breaking up with his girlfriend, and becoming more direct in his advances toward Meghan. She rejects all of them. He tells her, "I love you," and she says again how him favoring her like that was only undermining her ability to know whether she was actually good at her job. She turned him down, and he was humiliated.

"So I continued to do the cowardly thing, and I continued to do the selfish thing. Now, I wanted to teach her a lesson."

"That was probably the darkest of it all..." Harmon admits. "I said horrible things, just treated her cruelly, pointedly, things that I would never, ever, ever have done if she had been male... I lied to myself the entire time about it - and I lost my job (not because of the incidents, but from a larger breakdown in his life). "I ruined my show. I betrayed the audience. I destroyed everything. And I damaged her internal compass... And I moved on."

Here, Dan Harmon is describing the ***constriction*** *phase of healing where everything starts to fall apart as a result of the coping strategy (in his case, lying to himself). He is directly on his way to Confrontation - the confrontation with himself.*

"I never did it before, and I will never do it again, but I certainly wouldn't have been able to do it if I had any respect for women. On a fundamental level, I was thinking about them as different creatures. I was thinking about the ones that I liked as having some special role in my life. And I did it all by not thinking about it..."

"I want to say, I did it by not thinking about it - and I got away with it by not thinking about it. And if she hadn't mentioned something on Twitter, I would have continued to not have to think about it. Although, I did walk around with my stomach in knots about it. But, I wouldn't have had to talk about it."

~ ~ ~

"It was cathartic in a way that I could have never imagined", Ganz says about hearing his public apology while on her way to work. "I only listened because I expected an apology. But what I didn't expect was the relief I'd feel in hearing him say, '*These things actually happened*'."

During late 2017, in the wake of Harvey Weinstein and the #MeToo movement, Harmon tweeted, "This was truly the year of the asshole, myself included."

Dan Harmon told Nancy Updike, "Someone doesn't have to wish me harm to tell me that I harmed them."

He got advice from women in the business (note, not attorneys) and read a book his therapist recommended, *On Apology*, by Aaron Lazaar. "A complete apology has to start with an acknowledgment of offense.", the book reads. "i.e., wrenching your brain away from its justifications and putting yourself in the other person's place." Dan says, "It seems crucial that you not skimp there."

~ ~ ~

This is exactly what the men at modern-day Lawrence Academy were trying to do. They wanted to jump to the appearance-of-apology part without the acknowledgment-of-offense step. The line, *"We're not exactly in agreement about that"* was fed to me by Dan Scheibe before we even sat down for our (abbreviated) restorative process. They walked in fully armored, avoiding the most crucial piece in recovery for everyone: Honesty.

In 2020, Dan Scheibe, Paul Lannon, Bruce MacNeil, and Steve Hahn are still carrying that shield, despite all the dings of impact from me, alumni, the press, and families. The whole thing must be so tiring for them. To quote Anais Nin again, "When one is pretending, the entire body revolts." To pretend for this long, nearly four years since 'Asking People to Come Forward', must change a body entirely, to withstand the ongoing internal revolts.

This is how denial starts to weaken the one refusing to admit.

Dan Harmon then seems to have finally found the relief he was seeking. His voice has a sweet surrender as he says, "And I think that we're living in a good time right now because we're not gonna get away with it anymore." concluding his public apology.

"Dan's apology worked," says Nancy Updike, "partly because he finally took a risk - he admitted to things that, if Meghan had wanted, she probably could have used against him. Lawyers advised him to not say those things. By admitting them openly, **he chose her wellbeing over his own comfort**, maybe for the first time in their whole relationship."

~ ~ ~

"People who do very bad things, who have a lot of shame, who have a rickety platform of self-worth are entrenched non-apologizers.", says Harriet Lerner, author of the 2017 book, *Why Won't You Apologize?,* and the classics *The Dance of Anger* and *The Dance of Intimacy*.

"The non-apologizer walks on a tight rope of defensiveness, above a huge canyon of low self-esteem.", she says in a conversation with Brene Brown in 2020.

"I think for a lot of people, it will be counter-intuitive because it looks like non-apology is a function of arrogance and greatness.", Brown says.

"Well, what is arrogance?" Lerner asks.

"Right. Arrogance is low self-esteem." they agree.

"One of the things I found that was so shocking in my research," Brown continues, "the willingness to apologize and make amends was such a function of self-worth. The higher the self-worth, the higher the self-respect, the greater the willingness to apologize and make amends.

"So that when someone really does serious harm, and they don't have self-worth, and they have shame, if you confront them, they will really desperately justify and minimize and reverse the blame and even say, 'you caused it, you brought it upon yourself' or that it didn't happen, it never happened, [they will] invalidate the reality."

I certainly found all of this to be true in my wrangling with the men who make decisions at my former high school.

~ ~ ~

Can we love and accept ourselves when we mess up? Is it really all that fragile?

The Courage to Repair

I invited school leaders to a new Restorative Justice process in 2019 - one where Paul could not attend and "refute" my claims. Steve Hahn would have to stay for the 'making things right' conversation. We would have the full, necessary time. They denied every request.

Wed, May 29, 2019, 6:12 AM

to me, Dan

Dear Vanessa,

We are responding to your invitation for a second restorative justice process with the school. We appreciate and share your desire for a sound resolution, but we do not believe that a second meeting of this type would be helpful, given that we thoroughly engaged the process and all its components in our initial encounter. We have made our offers and positions clear in our previous communications.

Sincerely,

Bruce MacNeil
Dan Scheibe

Did he really believe that cancelling our Restorative Circle, leaving less than half the agreed-upon time, with no conclusion reached, and Steve Hahn leaving at lunch truly "thoroughly engaged the process and all its components"? Did Bruce MacNeil (who hadn't been present in any way) have the right to say that first effort was actually "good enough"?

It seemed to me, they simply wanted to have the final word on the matter (to the public) and end the conversation.

I Decline Your Offer As It Stands

June 4, 2019

Dan, Bruce,

I am writing to acknowledge your time-sensitive offer for financial settlement, expiring June 15, 2019.

Without an honest moment of admission, for the sake of recovery and growth, I cannot accept financial payout.

I am declining your offer as it stands. I am, as you know, seeking funding to support the Justice CORPS Initiative – to bring positive reform to the first two willing schools for the 2019-2020 school year. My current fundraising goal is $250,000, the minimum requirement to secure fiscal sponsorship through the nonprofit accelerator, Tides.

As a counter offer, I suggest that you apply $75,000 toward that effort. I have done all the work to register The Amends Project as a nonprofit in Washington state. Your donation would be greatly appreciated.

As for the conflict between the school and myself, I consider it unresolved. **Tenet # 4 of The Amends Project** states that the project only concludes "when leaders admit to the cover-up . . . and new policies are firmly in place to protect the rights and wellbeing of students for perpetuity." I accept that my goals may not be accomplished in this order.

Over these past two years of our active engagement, you have employed defamation, slander, dishonesty, denial cloaked as "disagreement", a duplicitous story, intimidation (do you really need that many police to try to arrest me at Open House?), disrespect for my limits, my time and more. These are your crimes. Choosing to dig in your heels on a stance of refusal to admit or to grow causes such harms...

As for your numbers – it occurs to me often that **nowhere in society does the defendant also get to be the judge**. Your opinion on your offer is of no substance to me. Secondly, if my former attorney, the undisputed expert in the field, concludes that we will reach a certain settlement – even before detailed documents surfaced – then I am sticking with that number.

With settlement, I seek the stability to continue my work of reforming schools to embrace transparency. I want this so that all kids can graduate high school safely and go on to begin their careers and achieve their aspirations sooner.

Again, I can only accept financial settlement that is accompanied by acknowledgement. **Honesty is what repairs.** You let me know when you are ready to proceed on that road.

In the meantime, here is the new fundraiser: [link]

Or, you may put donations directly into the nonprofit PayPal account: [link]

Truly,

Vanessa Osage

Jun 11, 2019, 1:04 PM

to me, Dan

Dear Vanessa,

Thank you for your reply. We are sorry that you are unable to accept our settlement offer in exchange for a release of claims. A donation to the Justice CORPS Initiative is not an alternative we can consider…

…we cannot provide the acknowledgement that you seek for allegations with which we fundamentally disagree. Primarily, we disagree that the school engaged in a cover up regarding Peter Regis' misconduct. The incident you brought to the school's attention was immediately reported, at that time, to the appropriate state authorities [*not to the police - which violated both law and school policy*]. While we have publicly acknowledged short-comings with the school's response, the matter was directly addressed both internally and externally [*what does that mean?*]. We also fundamentally disagree with your allegation that the school withdrew your financial aid or engaged in any other form of retaliation following your report.

Bruce MacNeil
Dan Scheibe

~ ~ ~

It was June 2019, when Bruce MacNeil finally admitted the nature of his "disagreement". They denied the cover up, and the choice to withdraw my financial aid. This was progress. It had been clear to me all along, yet intentionally unclear to others (even Sybil guessed they were disagreeing about my health issues being a consequence). He'd put it in writing. Clarity. One small step.

Remember former Lowell Sun Editor, Jim Campini's words, from June 4, 2018:

> "There's no doubt that a former Lawrence Academy administration conducted an egregious coverup and that present-day officials are trying to make amends. While the latter is laudable, the new regime seems reluctant to embrace transparency and accept responsibility for the sins of the past."

How could a group of men become so entrenched in a stance of denial, at such cost, for so long? What was Bruce MacNeil's role in the decision in the 1990s? He was a member of The Board of Trustees from 1984 onward. So, he was a key decision-maker at the time, as well.

Here is my biggest concern:

As they have left it today, the school's actions and public statements say to all without question, 'Disagree with our choices, or speak out against them, and there will be a price'. The message is: 'We will retaliate, then pretend it didn't happen, then chase you away for decades if you challenge us'.

Only when they say, "Punishing a child for speaking out is wrong, and we regret that choice", can the healing finally begin.

Jun 12, 2019, 8:51 AM

to Paul, Bruce, Dan

Bruce,

First, a responsible apology takes ownership of the choices made by the speaker. "I'm sorry *you*…", therefore, is always an avoidance of responsibility.

… Your belief in the lack of retaliation/cover-up serves only you. Your conclusion is not based in fact or reality, but in convenience.

… No lawyers or investigation, no carefully crafted language or lack of found evidence changes any of that. My lived experience is the ultimate testimony to what happened.

Unless, of course, you were instrumental in the decision to keep Pete Regis employed and to remove me. If so, it is time to speak up, Bruce. Otherwise, you will have to default to me as the authority in my own life.

… The Justice CORPS is necessary because there is a conflict of interest in protecting a school's reputation that continues to this day. I accept that Lawrence Academy will not participate in the program. Clearly, you're not ready yet for such a level of responsibility or trust in your kids and families. I am carrying on with progress elsewhere. Of course, donations are always optional.

I remain firm in my decision to turn down that offer as it stands.

Parent Letter

Once school was out for the summer of 2019, things were uncomfortably quiet.

I didn't know what to do now. Supporters had scattered into vacation plans, and the wave of social media attention rolled out, just as it had rolled in. When things seemed silent and hopeless, a letter arrived suddenly at my PO Box in Bellingham, Washington.

Dear Vanessa,

I am writing in reference to your June 10, 2018 Opinion piece in The Lowell Sun and The Amends Project.

Please find attached a copy of a letter sent to the Lowell Sun in 2017. The letter was written as part of an effort to make public sexual misconduct that occurred on the Lawrence Academy campus....

As I'm sure you're aware, one problem with Lawrence Academy's current approach of asking victims to come forward is that many victims do not want to relive their traumas. And many of the victim's parents do not want their professional reputations tarnished by unpleasant press about their daughters or sons. Many have accepted settlements and signed non-disclosures.

Achieving transparency on the campus of these private boarding schools is an uphill battle. They operate in a default mode of silence because silence preserves personal and professional reputations, high enrollments and increasing endowments. But if everyone agrees to keep things "confidential" the situation will not improve and lives will continue to be damaged.

I applaud your efforts to bring light to this topic and your *unwillingness* to be "bought" by the system that has silenced so many.

(unsigned)

The Lowell Sun

November 28, 2017

Subject: Lowell Sun story dated 10/22/2016 re: Lawrence Academy

[Remember, this was the "asking people with information to come forward" piece]

To Whom It May Concern:

On October 22, 2016, the Sun ran a story saying Lawrence Academy was asking people to come forward if they had information about sexual misconduct at the school. Lawrence Academy sent that request (in the form of a letter) to current families at the school, not to alumni or the families of alumni.

Dan Scheibe has a nephew, xxxx, who attended Lawrence Academy for his sophomore year and part of his junior year.

[this parent then outlines the familial relationship between the student and headmaster Dan Scheibe]

The two girls xxxx is alleged to have assaulted both graduated from Lawrence Academy. It is whispered that both girl's families were convinced by the school not to press charges or go to the police and were compensated for their silence. Some say their tuition was waived. Many past parents and students in the Lawrence Academy community know about these incidents. The identity of both of xxxx's victims is also widely known.

Shortly after xxxx had left the school a student awkwardly addressed the "xxxx incidents" in an All School Assembly, asking the question, "Why is it okay for the headmaster's nephew to do what he did and get away with it while those who commit more minor offenses are immediately expelled?" Some students at the school referred to xxxx as "the rapist".

Dan Scheibe seems to be a good headmaster who wants to do the right thing. Sending that letter encouraging people to report incidents of sexual assault was a positive thing and obviously an attempt to get out in front of the controversy that had embroiled so many other New England prep schools. It was a signal that Lawrence Academy had nothing to hide. But that letter was sent while his brother-in-law (Eric Peterson) was still embroiled in the sexual assault scandal at St. George's School that ultimately resulted in his resignation at the end of the academic year in 2017. And Eric Peterson's son (xxxx) had committed sexual assault at Lawrence Academy while Dan Scheibe was its headmaster.

If Scheibe were truly trying to surface incidents of sexual assault on his campus he'd have sent that letter to the fellow graduates of the girls his nephew has assaulted and to their parents. He chose not to do that. xxxx and Dan Scheibe need to be held accountable.

Wikipedia

"Wikipedia is a free online encyclopedia,
created and edited by volunteers around the world
and hosted by the Wikimedia Foundation."

Richard Rohr speaks in a conversation with Krista Tippett of OnBeing, about the long-view of human transformation, in what he calls a simplistic metaphor, of the three boxes: Order, Disorder, Reorder.

"That if you read the great myths of the world, and the great religions, that's the normal path of transformation. What conservative people want to do is just keep rebuilding the first box - order, order, order - at all costs, even if it doesn't fit the facts or fit reality.

"There's no non-stop flight from order to reorder. You've got to go through disorder. Your salvation project. It has to fall apart.

"What the great religions are talking about is the necessary confrontation with the tragic, the absurd... That disorder is part of the deal. That's so counterintuitive, I know.", Rohr says.

Tippet continues, "The moving from order to disorder to reorder... This is a choice each of us has. This trajectory to meaning, we are free to walk that path or not. It involves cross-over points, which involve, as you say, "necessary suffering", which is not something, as human creatures, we are drawn to do willingly. We often have to be kind of brought to our knees, it's moments of transition, it's moments of crisis, it's thresholds, it's facing our shadows.", Tippet says.

"There's no other way, Krista, the human ego will give up control - and hand over control - until it has to... It pretty much has to be forced onto us."

~ ~ ~

Dan Scheibe and Bruce MacNeil had the institutional authority to draw on the school's endowments to pay Paul Lannon, and his colleague Elizabeth Sanghavi, to create a controlled and safely revealing document. Then, they sought to shut it all down. Order, Order, Order. They had the law firm Holland & Knight and their associates. But, I had the creative commons. Disorder, and onward, to Reorder.

Whenever I would hit that point of seeming to reach a dead-end, I would ask myself, "What is the next, boldest thing I haven't thought of yet?"

Wikipedia.

I opened my first account and posted.

Soon, I found a notice on the internal dashboard titled, "Badly Written Scandal Section".

In it, the author complains about the section being "just so badly written" and protests my use of Pete Regis' name. I do further research to learn the restrictions for Wikipedia and edit my post so that it meets "Biographies of a Living Person" guidelines. I learned how to make citations, added these, and posted again.

Abuse Cover-up Scandal

Lawrence Academy played a role in the child abuse scandals at private boarding schools in the 1980s & '90's, by concealment of abuse on campus. Following two matching reports of child molestation in 1994, school officials chose to keep the accused person employed and living on campus. One of these students asked repeatedly what would be done, and was eventually told there was "no financial aid available for her return". She was prevented from attending the following year.

In 2016, Lawrence Academy headmaster Daniel Scheibe issued a public statement, asking people with information to come forward[9]. The former student who challenged their decision, Vanessa (Fadjo) Osage, '96, came forward, yet again. She had returned to the school annually, from 1994-2001, to insist on protection for incoming students; school officials were knowingly employing and housing a child molester. The member of staff was excused from employment seven years later, on "permanent long-term disability". The decision came when Ms. Osage was on her way to Groton, Massachusetts, at age 23, to give a speech in the Lawrence Academy auditorium on December 10, 2001[10]. He was released just days before her arrival. Then-headmaster Steven L Hahn resigned the following year.

In 2016, following the Boston Globe's Spotlight Investigation of Boarding Schools[11], Vanessa Osage retained attorney Mitchell Garabedian to represent her in a case against Lawrence Academy. In 2017, his office sent a demand letter to the school for $2 million in settlement. Soon after, Ms. Osage released the attorney, citing a mismatch of principles. She proceeded with resolution on her own. A feature article of her story was published in The Lowell Sun on May 27, 2018[12]. Following publication, nearly a dozen former students, parents and families contacted her with stories of cover-ups at Lawrence Academy, with some allegations as recent as 2017.

Lawrence Academy officials offered Ms. Osage 1% and then 3% of the attorney's demand, with a confidentiality clause, while "disagreeing" about what happened. She did not accept. Instead, she created a transparency and oversight model to prevent abuse cover ups called The Justice CORPS, the Committee to Oversee the Rights and Protections of Students[13], and incorporated her efforts into a state nonprofit called The Amends Project[14]. Lawrence Academy officials hired attorneys from Sanghavi Law Firm in the summer of 2018 to create a report, after more former students came forward with similar allegations. Elizabeth Sanghavi is a former associate of Holland & Knight[15], the law firm currently representing the school. Some former students proceeded with lawsuits. The academy released their findings in a report on April 25, 2019[16].

The report tallied four separate accounts of child molestation with students from 1991-1994. The scope of the investigation was outlined roughly as only covering incidents regarding the one former member of staff. This did not include the original two accounts given on campus in 1994. At least five impacted-former-students chose to not participate in the investigation. Ms. Osage asked for verification that the report would not be edited or abridged, and the school would not provide this.

The former students' accounts were found to be "credible", and school officials apologized publicly for the employee's behavior. Though, there has been no apology for the actions to cover up abuse. Another former student, "Student A" is cited in the report as saying, *"There was a backlash against the students who made the allegations, and the school did not address this".*

As of November 2019, school officials are yet to acknowledge the cover up behaviors, or to settle with Ms. Osage out of court.

~ ~ ~

Then, I found that the latest press on The Amends Project, the Lowell Sun piece with my quotes on their mistreating families to cover up abuse, was missing.

The link to the April 25, 2019 article now directed to a page that read, "Oops! That page can't be found.". I immediately called Kevin Corrado of Digital First Media, the parent company of The Lowell Sun. I did not get a call back. So, I emailed, asking that the story be replaced along with images to the Justice CORPS article. I looked and saw that all images had been removed from recent press on The Amends Project.

Many days passed, and I heard nothing. When I wrote again, I said I would file a complaint at the Federal level if I did not hear back by a certain date. Still, silence.

So, I contacted Lowell Sun Senior Editor, Tom Zuppa on August 20, 2019. Tom Zuppa wrote back, saying it had been a technical issue during a content management system switch and, "99.9% of stories had transferred over". This one simply had not. What are the chances?

He also called me "threatening" and said a simple request would have sufficed. Of course, numerous simple requests hadn't sufficed. So, reality cancelled that claim.

Here, we face the D's again - **Diversion**

If the major issue was my "threatening tone", then clearly, we didn't have to focus on the larger issue of journalistic integrity. Removing a news article from public access is a violation of public trust. What shall we focus on in this moment? **Diversion - Stay Focused**.

But, it all didn't stop there.

I did a search on Lawrence Academy - which I did from time to time - and saw all reference to The Amends Project and Lawrence Academy, this story, any press about me, or Pete Regis, or the report, was gone or many pages back in search results. It had been the third entry on Google for months. Then, it was gone. Somebody had cleaned up everything online.

I asked Tom Zuppa to send verification when the article was replaced, and he said he would. More time passed, with no confirmation.

I soon searched again and found a very similar article, marked as ***"updated"*** on August 21, 2019. The headline had been changed. A semi colon was added with the phrase, "school apologizes for response" following.

The alteration is captured in the hyperlinks:

https://www.lowellsun.com/breakingnews/ci_32596704/report-lawrence-academy-custodian-exposed-himself-students-1990s

https://www.lowellsun.com/2019/04/25/report-lawrence-academy-worker-exposed-himself-to-students-in-1990s-school-apologizes-for-response/

If I hadn't asked, this article would have remained out of sight entirely. Now it was back, but with a new and misleading message attached.

I contacted a number of employees at The Sun, and only one responded to say she couldn't reactivate the original story. I posted on The Amends Project page:

Year 2, Into Week 19: Goal # 1: Bring the Truth to Light

How many Lowell Sun employees does it take to reactivate an original, unaltered story?

No, it's not the set-up to a joke . . . *It's a question that shouldn't have to be asked.*

Complaint to the Federal Trade Commission – filed.

~ ~ ~

This was ridiculous. It was time to just call Tom Zuppa. What the hell was going on? I started searching for a phone number online, and instead, found this:

BOSTON BUSINESS JOURNAL

Senior editor at The Sun of Lowell suddenly leaves job[23]

By Don Seiffert – Managing Editor, Boston Business Journal
Aug 23, 2019, 12:53pm EDT

---

[23] Don Siefert, Boston Business Journal, August 23, 2019, https://www.bizjournals.com/boston/news/2019/08/23/senior-editor-at-the-sun-of-lowell-suddenly-leaves.html

Tom Zuppa, a 24-year veteran journalist at The Sun of Lowell, left his job yesterday as the paper's senior editor yesterday for what he says are "personal reasons."

Zuppa, who was a reporter at the Middlesex News (now called the MetroWest Daily News) for 15 years before joining the Sun as managing editor in 1995. He had just been named to the senior editor role in December 2018 by the Sun's parent company, MediaNews Group, which is owned by a hedge fund and formerly called Digital First Media.

Zuppa's departure came as a surprise to the newsroom, according to Sun insiders.

In a brief email to the Business Journal on Friday morning, Zuppa confirmed that he had left, but didn't elaborate on the reasons behind the decision.

I called The Boston Business Journal and spoke to Don Sieffert, the reporter. I was shaking when I dialed the number. It so clearly reeked of a dodge from accountability move. Don Sieffert was polite and curious; he asked me to follow up with an email.

He and I then went back and forth over days and weeks. I asked him to look into it. He said it seemed unlikely to be connected. He asked for suggestions on how to get to the bottom of it. I sent specific ideas on people to contact at The Sun, Digital First, and Lawrence Academy and provided contact information. He didn't follow up on any of them. Instead, he said he would ask Tom Zuppa again.

Notice the power play: a reporter says, "Tell me what to do." A concerned citizen gives specific instructions. The reporter ignores these. Then, he repeats a previous move with the same results and claims defeat. I later regretted, and pointed out, my effort to essentially do part of his job while he ignored potential sources. Was this sincerely not a strong lead?

I thought an Accreditation Director would care deeply about evidence of one of its verified schools covering up child abuse on campus. I met resistance and soon, criticism. I thought a reporter would care deeply about evidence of an altered headline coinciding with an Editor's sudden, unexplained resignation. I met a mysterious lack of willingness to act. Both attempted to redirect me elsewhere. Both seemed to see little reason for concern.

Yet, I will continue to see a need for reorienting this all to the upright and above-board. Sage wisdom I once overheard encouraged, simply, "If it doesn't make sense, don't accept it.". That move helps us hold the line to common sense when other forces might tip things sideways.

I will continue to care about righting and clarifying and orienting civic life toward values of truth and justice. Why? *You find what you put out there.*

I updated the Wikipedia entry to include the latest unfolding regarding Tom Zuppa and the changed headline.

"The former students' accounts were found to be "credible", and school officials apologized publicly for the employee's behavior. Though, there has been no apology for the actions to cover up abuse. Another former student, "Student A" is cited in the report as saying, *"There was a backlash against the students who made the allegations, and the school did not address this".*

The Lowell Sun continued press coverage[17] on Lawrence Academy and The Amends Project from May 2018 to April 2019. In September 2019, Lowell Sun Managing Editor, Tom Zuppa, suddenly left his job[18] after discovery of alteration of the most recent online article on the story. A phrase, ";school apologizes for response" was added to the headline, months after publication. A complaint has been filed with the Federal Trade Commission.

As of November 2019, school officials are yet to acknowledge the cover up behaviors, or to settle with Ms. Osage out of court."

~ ~ ~

Over the next few weeks, at the start of the school year, I would find the entry completely removed without cause. I commented that I was willing to consider specific complaints or suggestions - but taking it down entirely was a violation.

There was no response to this, so for many days, I simply made it part of my morning routine. Like brushing my teeth. I'd go to the computer, replace what had been removed, and go about my day.

Soon, there was a "disruptive editing" complaint.

I contacted Wikipedia to make my own complaint:

Hello,

I am writing to make a complaint of an inappropriate block. There is a level of harassment involved, as well.

I have been adding factual, relevant, very well cited information to the History section of this page: https://en.wikipedia.org/wiki/Lawrence_Academy_(Groton,_Massachusetts)?action=edit

The harassment has appeared in the form of vague insults within messages "it's just so badly written..." and continual removal of the information. It is clearly designed to intimidate me into not replacing the information.

The term "disruptive editing" may be a more accurate description of the user removing the section without due cause. I have carefully read the Wikipedia guidelines on "Biographies of a Living Person" and removed names and all unnecessary adjectives.

Lawrence Academy of Groton, MA does not control wikipedia. They are attempting to hide important information about the ways in which they have hidden abuse. I also filed a police report last year for bullying, after they attempted to arrest me on campus at an Open House event.

Please take to heart that this institution has a clear record of trying to bully people into silence about their mistakes.

Again, all references have been documented – either by real newspaper articles, live audio and/or external websites.

I ask that officials at Wikipedia take action to prevent the blocking of information – especially as it relates to child safety at our public service institutions.

This fight for "control of the story" continued throughout September and heightened in the days leading up to their next Open House event. I noticed the date for Open House that year was not posted anywhere on the Lawrence Academy website. I speculated that this was an attempt to hide from unwanted attention. Knowing that prospective families had a good chance of searching the school online leading up to the event (and finding the fuller story there) became its own practical reward.

Of course, Wikipedia is consensus-based. So, if one administrator with something to hide disagrees with a post, it can ultimately be blocked.

For my last update to Wikipedia I described my changes this way:

Edit Summary (briefly describe your changes)

Replaced relevant, accurately cited information. Because bullying takes many forms and wears many guises. Some may believe there are benefits in acting so - but suppressing important truths isn't one of them.

White Male Privilege: Q & A

That web of complacency, hiding, secrecy, refusing to investigate, and all of the ways 'men in power' sought to block the truth of this started to feel very dark. September 2019 was also the time of "Sharpie-gate" when Donald Trump took a sharpie pen to an official map of the projected path of Hurricane Dorian. This altered document, he held up for the country to see. He did it to match evidence to a false comment he'd made on Twitter, that the storm could hit the state of Alabama. It was a simple mistake, for which he could have quickly apologized and offered clarification. But, no.

The National Weather Service had to come in twenty minutes later and post, "Alabama will NOT see any impacts from #Dorian. We repeat, no impacts from Hurricane #Dorian will be felt across Alabama. The system will remain too far east."

For my own healing, I tried out a new form of writing. I just needed to make myself laugh. I posted it on Medium:

White Male Privilege: Q & A

White Male Privilege, or WMP, is now being recognized as a social disease by psychologists and experts in the field of public health. The Center for Social Diseases, CSD*, has released these guidelines for understanding, diagnosing and treating White Male Privilege.

How common is White Male Privilege?

White Male Privilege affects about 28% of the United States population, with higher concentrations in the urban epicenters of New York, Boston and Los Angeles.

How do I know if I have White Male Privilege?

Diagnosis occurs as distorted thinking that presents as a **"cluster of symptoms"**. The disease can affect both individuals and institutions or groups where the cluster of symptoms is present, taught or shared. WMP can be contagious, with short or long-term exposure to those suffering from the disease increasing the incidence. There is currently no conclusive test to confirm or rule out the disease.

Wait, I am white and male, does that mean I have White Male Privilege?

No. Fortunately, characteristics do not indicate causality. One can be white and male without being infected by the cluster of symptoms that indicate presence of the disease.

Resistance to social pressure and a diverse world view have been strongly correlated with preventative factors. Knowing and loving people who do not live a privileged experience has also been shown to reduce the incidence. Researchers have gathered inspired stories of individuals resisting the pull of the disease, even when surrounded by it.

The CSD has identified the following list of Ten Telltale Symptoms:

1. You believe you are superior to other people, and exempt from the rules governing regular society. When you encounter a limit that does not support your desires or view of yourself, you conclude that it simply doesn't apply. You may have excessive debt, lawsuits or unpaid penalties against you.

2. You might enjoy the rush of "special circumstances" such as favors or access to things denied to others, only to suffer a crushing guilt of believing you are unworthy, and subsequent anxiety over getting caught.

3. You have an explosive reaction to feedback, and an unchecked urge to blame others until you feel relief and comfort again.

4. You have irrational fears of women (if you are a heterosexual male, this can coexist as simultaneous attraction/fear) as well as people of color, LGBTQ and gender nonconforming people.

5. You lack trust in those who do not look like you, yet also feel trapped by not really trusting your White Male Privilege friends either. You are lonely because of a constant worry that you will be excluded from the club.

6. You resent your dependence on human beings and hoard excess resources to feed an illusion of 'not needing others'. You believe that, 'In life, there are winners and losers, and it's ok to create losers to ensure that you are a winner; That's just the way it is.'

7. You have an intense urge to control others, which you may perceive as simply being "strong", "decisive" or "dominant". You may have heard from friends and loved ones that they feel misunderstood by you, but you see this as their weakness and not your problem.

8. You have made, or are making, decisions to protect your reputation or financial assets at the expense of other people. Your belief in your superiority has allowed you to justify these choices. Yet, deep down, you feel even more inadequate because you know no other way to 'play the game and win'.

9. You might believe that women or young people owe you access to their bodies, or that the unpaid/underpaid work of 'lesser' people is your birthright to enjoy. You often feel lonely, yet can't imagine why.

10. Your behavior is increasingly destructive, and you feel further and further from your own sense of right and wrong. You are caught in a cycle of hurting

others, seeking to feel better about yourself through superiority, and then feeling even worse. Your relationships suffer, and then your physical health weakens without apparent explanation.

Experts say that any combination of four or more of the above symptoms is considered a WMP diagnosis. Six or more symptoms is a severe case of White Male Privilege. WMP is a progressive disease, and early intervention is the key to effective treatment.

What are the risk factors?

WMP can be hereditary and occurs more often in families where the cluster of symptoms is passed on or even praised from a distance.

Exposure to generational or family financial wealth has been shown to increase the incidence of White Male Privilege. Though, again, this factor alone is not causational.

Interestingly, those who began life with very little resources can be highly susceptible to developing the disease later in life. Anyone who has felt particularly low about themselves or their life situation — and has not reconciled these feelings — could fall prey to its influence at some point.

Men with a criminal record, or something to hide, can be more inclined to adopt one or more of the symptoms. The distorted thinking of being 'above others' may offer pointed relief to those already carrying a burden of guilt over poor choices in their past.

Lastly, anyone who was confronted with the experience of acute anxiety and lack of control as a child is at higher risk. When pain and control coexist over time, distorted thinking can occur. Case studies have revealed that early fears were at the root of some of the most severe cases. ***Letting boys be scared and giving them a supportive space to work through their fears is encouraged.***

What if I love someone affected by White Male Privilege? What can I do?

Those living in proximity with WMP patients can be affected in a number of ways. Loved ones need to watch for the negative effects of gaslighting, discrediting and dismissal coming from WMP sufferers. Relationships are especially hard for those with White Male Privilege, and new research is currently being done to understand the brain and hormonal chemistry of those affected.

The best approach is to get help by connecting with people who do not suffer from WMP, while finding the strength to hold WMP sufferers accountable for their actions at every step. Pretending or going along only aggravates the disease and delays recovery.

The Center for Social Diseases expects new 12-Step Programs and support groups to pop up in highly affected areas, following release of these findings.

Like other addictions, WMP can be a progressive disease. Self-care must be a priority for those living in proximity to the disease. Loved ones are encouraged to only maintain connections that include strong boundaries and to adopt a stringent practice of truth-telling in the presence of WMP sufferers. Be ready to endure child-like tantrums, and to hold firm while telltale behaviors present themselves. Remember, "keeping them honest" is an act of love.

Patience and compassion are needed, as WMP sufferers are often overly scared, fragile and unsure of themselves. Go slowly but remain firm. They may seem to enjoy special privileges, but remember, they are suffering.

I think my boss or other public figures suffer from WMP, what should I do?

It is important to not feed any illusion that those with WMP are special or above others. Unfortunately, they do often find themselves in positions of authority because of an attraction to *telltale-symptom-affirming cultures*.

At times, the bravado of developed WMP sufferers can lure some into a false sense of security. It is important to think long-term and remember that **the**

one who does not need to put others down is always the stronger candidate. Our most effective and beloved leaders have an innate appreciation of the ills of WMP (regardless of race, gender, orientation or identity) and see inherent value in the lives and experiences of all.

Simple actions, such as respecting others' limits, asking permission, saying 'I'm sorry' and 'Thank you' have shown promise as a path to rewiring the brains of early WMP sufferers. Cutting edge research is now underway.

Resisting White Male Privilege on the social, economic and political levels is its own practice of recovery. Keep in mind, the population was infected long-ago, when the disease was still largely unseen and unidentified.

We can all help normalize shows of humanity, compassion, valuing a diversity of life, and the humility that keeps everyone honest in everyday interactions. This social norming can be a part of the slow and necessary cultural transformation.

Is there a cure?!

Curing White Male Privilege is going to take a concerted effort by everyone affected by and surrounding its negative impacts in society.

As a public health crisis, it is our civic duty to interrupt White Male Privilege whenever we see it in a way that is consistent, loving and firm.

Remember, truth-telling, holding sufferers accountable and rejecting the ill-effects will help curb the spread of the disease. Only cooperation and a commitment to dismantling White Male Privilege (and its support structure, Patriarchy) will allow for social healing to occur.

Visit https://theamendsproject.com for a solution, and to learn more.

*This story is an illuminating spoof, and no such Center for Social Diseases, CSD, exists. Though, WMP and its effects, are real.

Male Initiation - Humanizing

Father Richard Rohr speaks of his decades of research into rites of passage globally, "That on every continent, culture after culture, it was never assumed that the young male naturally grew up (laughs warmly). He had to be taught. He had to be carefully taught... That was called initiation.

"Basically, here was the assumption that cultures came to - and at this point, I don't think it needs much proof - that unless the male was led on journeys of powerlessness, he would always abuse power. And I know that seems damning. But, the male just can't handle power unless he's somehow touched upon vulnerability, powerlessness. And it's no surprise, that that's the first step of the 12-Step Program.

"An important part of every initiation rite was grief work. Letting men get in touch with their unfinished hurt and begin to talk about it to other men. That's when the floodgates opened. And all of this success that they shine with externally, they finally could admit was all a charade.

"Everything changed after that."

~ ~ ~

When I led groups of young women into the wilderness for their solo overnight vigil, as a rite of passage from childhood into adolescence, a profound shift took place in them before their departure. Whatever fears or doubts they'd been holding all rose to the surface, and each had the chance to work with them in a structured way. Life got real. Some got focused and task-oriented, telling me what they would need and asking for assistance. Some clung to their friends. Some went inward and drew on a strength I couldn't see until we met them in the morning, glowing from the test endured.

When we hide from the tests of life or seek to prevent a test at all, we stunt our growth and wither into lesser versions of ourselves. The classic male initiation has involved military training to shut down the emotional, responsive parts of men and women to enact violence: going to war. A real rite of passage strengthens us. We know now that war only breaks men, women, families and countries. We need new rites of passage - and the opportunities lay out before us.

In elite or religious institutions, many are avoiding the true tests life brings. When faced with abusive behavior by teachers, priests or students, an authority must draw a line for health and reassert shared values in action. Transparency, care, and protection are the highest expression of masculine strength here. The Justice CORPS leads men (and decision-makers of any gender) into journeys of powerlessness by removing the ability to control outcomes. Humans in pain are not meant to be controlled or silenced.

This reform model faces the fact that a problem exists - and the problem grows and amplifies when avoided. The Justice CORPS, as a systemic overhaul, puts the power of response into other hands. It allows the messy, awkward, humane response to unfold naturally so healing can occur. All of this lashing out by school leaders with defamation, "lawyering up", silencing, controlling the story - it is the panic before the overnight vigil. This cultural reckoning moment is the initiation and these 'leaders' must walk into the wilderness alone to face what lies within and without.

We can't slink back into the comfort of control or false statements as a culture. We have to face this dark night to see the sunrise on the other side.

While lawsuits are often the best choice for many, they prevent the long-range goal of reform because the process encourages both hiding and violence. If clients are never allowed to speak to one another, and attacking the opponent is standard procedure, we just keep sliding back and back.

Humbly facing each other is how we transform. Handling each other with the strength in our humanity is how we heal.

Humanizing means holding leaders accountable by calling out the behavior (corruption) while calling in the person before us. There are universal sensitivities, strengths, weaknesses, confusions, and longings in the forces that move in all of us. We have to meet courageously on that ground. No one will be compelled from a place of "you are evil" to the willingness to see a fuller reality and create new solutions. Those forces move in opposite directions.

We go in fighting, because there are layers of defenses to get through to reach the tender, fertile place. We fight to disturb the stagnation that has built up behind the shields of self-defense. We can break down the shield in intentional or unexpected moments. Ideally, we arrive at the honest, tender place together. Then, we have to take a breath and bare our hearts.

There will be tension.

Too much tension - among opposing sides, motivations, or driving forces - results in some kind of a break, either violent or simply destructive. Too little tension, and nothing is challenged - no interplay, no engagement, or positive change will occur.

We must be willing to evoke and create those tensions. We are changed by the dance. So, we have to start moving and being moved. We can play with the tensions along the way. But, the ultimate point of transformation will always arrive through humanizing.

~ ~ ~

Padraig O'Tuama is the former leader (2014-2019) of the Corrymeela Community, Ireland's oldest peace and reconciliation community. It was formed in the wake of violent fracture and war in Northern Ireland, in the 1960's. The center won a Nobel Peace Prize in 1997, the year before the Good Friday Agreement brought an official end to war in the country. In a conversation with Krista Tippett, O'Tuama talks about the scale of sectarianism. He references work done by Cecelia Clegg and Joe Liechty, who say that Sectarianism is *belonging gone bad.*

O'Tuama describes, "The scale for them begins — I think there's about 14 or 15 points. The first part of the scale is going, "You're different. I'm different. Fine." And the 15th point is, "You're demonic."

Tippett adds, "And the farther down that scale you go, the more violence..."

O'Tuama continues, "The more danger. Yeah. The more you justify it, because if somebody is the devil, well, then you get rid of them, generally. One of the scales is, "In order for me to be right, it is important that I believe that you are wrong."

Mitchell Garabedian had said to me in 2016, "What they did to you was evil." And I recoiled from the speaker of the word evil. I spoke with another attorney in 2019 about suing current Lawrence Academy administrators for legal violations incurred since I came forward again in 2016.

The attorney said, quoting Theodore Roosevelt, "If you've got them by the balls, their hearts and minds will follow.", and laughed.

I have to disagree. You might be able to get results that way in the short-term. But what happens when you let go? You've got someone right beside you, with a personal vendetta to settle. You have scared someone into submission, so you get the chain reaction of consequences of harmful force.

What I know is that people make bad decisions when they're scared. I would choose a population of calm, clear, secure people over fearful ones any day. No matter the shared context or purpose. Roosevelt also said, "Walk softly and carry a big stick.". More than a few people have used this expression to describe me and how I move in the world.

"Walk softly and carry a big stick", to me, means being gentle, warm and loving in nature - yet bold, fierce and daring in actions.

With so much breaking down in our world now, it is time to daringly reimagine who we could be. Have the restrictions of gender and power halted all of us in our evolution? Men of many generations have been asked to violate their humanity for the sake of proving a social status that would confirm their manhood. Nobody's manhood should be on the line for the failure to act out a form of violence. I believe in a golden masculine, an exalted feminine, and the myriad of expressions therein, that allows us to be all of who we are.

My rejection of patriarchy is a prayer for what we can all be, in the next highest expression of our humanity. I see an entire ecosystem yearning for our evolution. I hear the cry as an insistence that will not yield until we finally respond with the courage of change.

~ ~ ~

The benefits of privilege are tenuous and unreliable.

The game of patriarchy has now started to self-destruct, coming undone by its weak internal links. Who defines who is on the inside and who is on the outside? Is that person eternally safe? No. When one is unsafe, all others instinctively sense they could be next. This is why Bruce MacNeil '*shoots the school in the foot*' when he unapologetically defames me to the press. That move sends a ripple of fear through the hearts of parents, who wonder how their child might be treated if they spoke up about abuse.

You just can't isolate one cruelty from another. You may believe you are on the 'inside' circle. Surely, if it were your child, they would support and protect you... *Maybe. But, maybe not.* With everything kept behind closed doors, loyalties could fall off a known edge in a secret meeting and go unseen by any caring eyes for decades or more. Time to come out from hiding. Transparency is the solution. Only integrity can satisfy our hunger for a world that makes sense.

Parents-as-consumers can insist on higher safety standards, and schools-as-suppliers will have to respond. The market must always meet the demand.

The pressures that arise for school leaders following abuse - we know from history - can have terrible, unexpected consequences. A seemingly "good" person will do or say unethical things. Consider headmaster Dan

Scheibe and his perceived regard for students in contrast to his choices. The decision-making currently rests in the wrong hands. It is our job as parents, advocates, concerned citizens, and members of adult society to wrestle that power out of those hands and place it elsewhere.

We have to admit that things have gotten bad enough that a root level response is necessary. Over 300 incidents at over 100 schools. Thousands in the Church. We have reached and passed the bad-enough point. Privilege, like masculinity, has precarious rules for inclusion. Tragically, patriarchy has dictated that "manhood" is also conditional and revocable. These are too many internal pressures on school officials. With such tenuous threads holding up our leaders, they are simply not steady enough to make the right choice when it matters. Other people, in other positions, can do so without bias or pressure.

It might be the most humane thing we can do for everyone involved.

Useful Skills - Staying With It

"Can you fight the urge to run for another day?
You might make it further,
if you learn to stay."

— Brandi Carlile

"There is no need to be ashamed of tears,
for tears bear witness
that a man has the greatest of courage,
the courage to suffer."

—Viktor Frankl

Staying With It is the fierceness of presence that Angeles Arrien speaks of in *The Four Fold Way* and also endurance.

Arrien says, "The principle that guides the Warrior is choosing to show up and be present." That means being present to what is true. Once a truth is fully seen, outside of the speaker and the listener, the alchemy of transformation begins. We have to evolve our notions of punishment and notions of power into a fierce willingness to see ourselves, and not flinch, not deny, not look away. But to stay with it until it transforms.

Men of certain generations or social classes have received a message that they 'don't have to deal' with emotional, interpersonal situations. I've watched comfortable, affluent New England men in particular attempt to signal to a group that they are above shows of emotional upset. They disengage and pretend they are too manly for such "soft" things. Husbands delegate to wives, fathers distance from sons and daughters, and the shutting down begins.

I now recognize this as posturing. *'I don't have to deal with this'* becomes, *'I don't know how to deal with this'*, which in essence is, *'I am scared because I have no skills to deal with this and still feel safe'*. It is a disempowered stance. You might say it is the opposite of being a warrior. Research shows that men are more easily "flooded" by negative emotion than women (80% more of the time)[24], and take longer to regulate their system after flooding occurs. Combining physiology with negative social conditioning leaves whole generations of us reeling in the wake of men's "not dealing" behaviors.

Staying With It is a new kind of warrior strength - one required of each of us now. Staying with difficult emotions may be the test for some. Staying with your faith in humanity and personal resilience is the goal for another. Staying with the courage to express your dissatisfaction and allow a minor conflict to play out is a different kind of triumph. You'll know what your challenge currently is if you are honest with yourself.

A few years ago, my guide in Restorative Justice, Saroeum Phoung, accepted the challenge of working with a Seattle teen who was facing jail time. Over an intense year-long process of owning a mistake, talking about what led to the arrest, offering public apologies and reparations, the two built trust. Saroeum says of the teenager, "The first time we sat down together, he told me, 'I don't like sharing things with strangers, and this is something I feel ashamed of.' What people don't realize is that this restorative justice work is harder than going to jail!"

---

24 https://www.johngottman.net/wp-content/uploads/2011/05/Physiological-and-affective-predictors-of-change-in-relationship-satisfaction.pdf

That is the power of Staying With It.

I remember how hard it was, even impossible at times, to stay with the pain of institutional abuse and retaliation. It took years for me to build strength to even allow the feeling, and stay with it... until it could shift. Nothing changes when we ignore it. We grow a new layer of wisdom when we are strong enough to keep looking at it, open ourselves to understanding it, and heartily respond. Healing is feeling and then dealing. We don't get to skip the first two steps.

~~~

For endurance, I've found two primary lines of strength: purpose and perspective.

Once we know what we are here to do, that resonance moves us in powerful ways. We can be here for multiple reasons in a lifetime. Whatever that purpose may be, anything that would throw you off track is less important than the track itself. We commit to the path we walk, and how we walk it, and life rewards us with vitality and a sense of rightness. Then, the universe responds with synchronicities, supportive coincidences to encourage that path along.

Perspective has repeatedly helped me to keep that commitment. Connection with elders has always been a source of uplifting perspective for me, beginning with my grandmother. From the vantage point of later life, one more easily sees what is most important. I revel in the chance to share that sight by proximity and care of elders.

A low point for me in the journey to institutional reform with Lawrence Academy was a phone call I made to a mother on the Parents Association. I had been reaching out to everyone I could think of, to advance The Justice CORPS Initiative and bring transparency to the system. I always figured parents would be most invested in seeing this change take hold. One mother picked up and calmly, curiously engaged the conversation. She said,
~~~

"If cover-ups are happening now, I would definitely be interested in hearing more.". She was the most supportive and receptive parent.

On the other extreme, though, was a mother full of fear. What surprised me was that she wasn't scared about potential injustice or retaliation for her child; she was scared of me. When I said why I was calling, she interrupted with a panic, *"Is this the victim?!"*. There was that word again. I said, "I am definitely more of an advocate at this point..." She described how upset she'd been over what school leaders told about my plans to ruin her son's graduation. Remember my call for attendees to wear yellow? Clearly, school officials had interjected a unique spin on who I was and what I set out to do.

It broke my heart to hear a parent respond to me in fear. I had built a vast network of trust in my professional career over the previous decade. That trust was graciously given to me by parents, school leaders, young adults, and children. In my work, I held sacred, tender things for so many in confidence, supporting people of all kinds in meaningful ways. Hearing a mother's voice responding to me in fear was both jarring and devastating.

To return to endurance after that kind of defamation required perspective. Given what Bruce MacNeil had said about me to the Lowell Sun, it wasn't hard to imagine what they might write to parents (in an effort to invalidate my message and protect their reputations). I had to keep sight of the goal. The vision of lasting justice and safety could pull me through. I knew what mattered.

When I am 90+ years old, will it matter what Bruce MacNeil or Dan Scheibe said about me to the press or parents behind my back? No. What will matter is the child who is less lonely or afraid because a woman came and spoke the previously unspeakable. Someone will be brought back into hope and vitality because they got the message they deserve better than institutional abuse. That liberation will matter.

In a distant way, I sometimes imagine a final turning point of this life and the emotional quality of what will remain. If I keep making wise trade-offs, shedding old ways for new, what will ultimately be worth it?

~ ~ ~

In the weeks after giving birth at 30 years old, I adjusted to motherhood and a world without my Gramma in it. I held that amazing new life at my chest, and it all seemed so obvious - the point, the purpose, and the enduring perspective. Gramma had been all about love. There were surface things that were uniquely her: the time in which she grew, how she responded, her style and humor, her challenges, and triumphs.

My Gramma lived into her 90s. She could remember the advent of the automobile, the fight for women's suffrage, and a time when *phones* required a switchboard operator. Her mother taught her to "count to ten in indian" on their southern California homestead, over a hundred years ago. She saw the shape of a world I can only imagine.

From time to time, I like to envision how she might see the world I see today. Her gaze lives on in me - her granddaughter, who had to outrun and outlive the ill-effects of a patriarchal system. Running and enduring to a personal triumph out past her lifetime. Most of all, Gramma was fiercely committed to living by love. I feel it coursing through me even now, like a river that brings everything sacred in a lifetime. Her perspective still sets the world back to upright.

If God says, "you must kill your son to please me," and man says, "ok," maybe we've got it all wrong. When doing the right thing is considered 'unreasonable', when cruelty is encouraged in private, yet scorned in public, we are too far off track. When leaders try to control perceptions instead of cultivating a healthy reality, the world starts to tip upside-down. You might not dream of a house ripped from its foundation and spinning in the air, but you've probably felt the dizziness at some point in your life.

Only when we drop anchor into a bedrock of love, truth and integrity can the topsy-turvy right itself again. No exceptions for certain people. No tolerance for false public statements. No celebrated cruelty or injustices. We can restructure our systems now and rethink the concepts that shaped these stories long ago.

Maybe the destruction around us, from institutionally-backed child abuse to racial violence, environmental degradation, and economic injustice... maybe it's all signs of the old story dying. Those values have played themselves out to the point that even their echo bounces off the remnants of decay. Yet, we do not have to let the best of ourselves die with it. Everything is a choice.

Remember, staying hopeful in the face of corruption is an act of defiance.

You find what you put out there.

Own it.

~ ~ ~

I think back to Sister (our lady of Kindness) from Catholic grade school in Massachusetts. She said to me when I was eleven years old, “You march to the beat of a different drummer.”. Thoreau said, “Let him step to the music which he hears, however measured or far away...”.

I do hear a rhythm.

Steady and strong, it’s a drum like a heartbeat.

A heartbeat like a song.

All these voices ringing out now, "Me Too", "My generation is watching. How dare you?!", "Black Lives Matter", they are the passerine songbirds at sunrise, calling in a new day. It has been dark, but I hear them all singing out now, in robust and more intricate chorus as the light grows brighter around us...

Louder now.

Here it comes.

Lucid Dream Road

By fall of 2019, the frantic energy of public attention rolled away like showers of lightning in a thunderstorm. The ground was quiet but electric, and I could feel the season change.

I had another quick exchange with Jamie Baker. I left her a voicemail, and she responded via text message. She said she was no longer at Lawrence Academy, by Dan Scheibe's decision, and she now had her own legal battles with the school. I was shocked yet again at what felt like the same dark energy reaching into the lives of people I cared about - pain that was not transformed but transferred.

That evening, I pondered on divergences again. People were moving away from old ways of doing things, sometimes parting ways, pulled by magnetic force toward growth and integrity. If Steve Hahn, Dan Scheibe, Bruce MacNeil, and Paul Lannon were now repelling people like Jamie Baker, too, how would this thing transform?

The leaves were falling, and the air grew cold outside. One thought kept coming back to me, over and over again:

I don't have faith in them, but I have faith in something.

~ ~ ~

It all reminded me of a different fall evening fifteen years earlier, in northern New Mexico.

My earliest years of traveling often felt like lost time - or life out of time. I would enter extended, relaxed mental states similar to meditation. There were times, from there, when I faced existential questions that echoed of fear and pain. They were questions that deserved to be asked all the same. What was there to keep me tethered to this world when truth and goodness were punishable offenses?

Notions like clouds would form shapes and dissolve overhead, as I drifted down the river of my new life, post-leaving home. Out beyond the edge of not coming back, I'd floated past the raw and disturbing idea of no one knowing where I was. Did it ever matter again what happened to me? And what of caring? What was there to hold any of us steady where we were, and how would I recognize it?

It turns out there was something.

So, I arrived at a unique juncture on a late fall afternoon in northern New Mexico, about nine years after leaving home. By then, I traveled only the blue highways - the smaller, lesser-known roads of America. These are the truer paths to traverse a landmass - the same way the details of a face, or a life, or even a global system, tell the fuller story. In these years, I still longed to travel the roads of this country, but with less urgency and often more bliss.

I'd noticed the place on my large paper atlas of New Mexico where the road simply changed color. Only, to my surprise, the road ended there. It felt like a joke, as if I'd suddenly found Shel Silverstein's *Where the Sidewalk Ends*. The pavement literally ran out, and my wheels rolled onto the gravel of a smudged path pointing up a long, winding incline. I couldn't see much beyond that point. The sun would be going down soon, and I hadn't seen signs of civilization for maybe two hours.

Somehow, I decided there was no going back.

I drove a late-model Isuzu Trooper in those days, with 4-wheel-drive and a sturdy frame above excellent vehicle clearance. This was just a new kind of adventure, I told myself. I put it into 4-wheel-drive and blazed ahead. The first hours were easy, while I was energized by the novelty and a newfound confidence. It was my tenth trip across the country. I could do this.

The light was disappearing, and a blanket of darkness unrolled at my feet, setting a whole new tone to my journey. Now, it was sincere and undeniable. I would not see sunlight again that day, and no outer lights of any kind lit this path. I met that vast wilderness with a focused, somber gaze. At one point after sunset, I pulled over and stepped out to pee. The quiet of the landscape was an immense presence around me. My breathing sounded louder than I'd ever heard, and a cricket moving in a dry bush echoed a gale force back to me. The sky was speckled with infinite layers of stars in natural finery like I had never seen.

I understood this was not a path to sleep along or beside. I didn't know how long it would even remain a discernible path. It was more defined in some places than others. Only one car passed me early on, heading in the opposite direction at twilight. Headlights had approached from above, and a vast dust cloud lingered behind both of our trails. I would have to make it all the way to the other side of this pass, to whatever lay beyond.

The narrow beam of my headlights illuminated a stark contrast to the blackness in all directions. Trees gave way to brush as I climbed higher and higher in elevation. Soon, I could see nothing but what was right in front of me.

Then, I met absurdity as an entry point to the divine.

Suddenly, a jackrabbit darted across the beam of light. That got my attention, and I sat up straighter in my car's bucket seat. Long limbs like a photograph of light lingered in my eyes. Then, another. Soon, these rabbits populated the light beam at a rapidly increasing rate. A flash of pale movement illuminated my view now, every 10 - 40 seconds. I couldn't believe the amount of rabbits!

I'd heard the jokes about rabbits and reproduction, but this seemed unreal. For a moment, it was absurdly funny and I laughed in exhilaration. It felt like being in a video game, with me clenching the wheel and turning abruptly to avoid them. The Isuzu was boxy and tall, which was great for sleeping in and navigating the snow, but terrible for quick turns away from jackrabbits. It felt like one sudden jerk of the wheel could knock the thing over.

Sometimes, two appeared together in tandem, or they'd come from different sides and barely staggered. I slowed to a crawl of maybe 30 mph, knowing all the while my need for sleep was only increasing. The humor receded into concentration. I soon settled into the middle of this path (I hadn't seen another car for many hours) to have the widest swerving margins. It was game-on.

It also bears mentioning: I had a long succession of pet rabbits as a child. Soft, domesticated creatures that lived in a hutch in the backyard, braving year-round New England weather. So, I felt a real kinship and affinity with rabbits. These were wilder, long-limbed, feral beings in their natural element of a desolate mountain pass. Somehow, I loved these even more fiercely in my own wild heart.

The disbelief faded, and soon, it was pure, clear focus. I had to get through this. I didn't know how long it would go on, but I was alert and single-minded. I felt my caring - and what truly drove me through the bizarre maze was clear-eyed determination. I was so utterly alone out there. The task seemed meaningful and also maybe insignificant. It was the value of every single life right there juxtaposed with the vastness of the universe. What fell away, and what could stay? Did I really have agency in how many of these animals would survive?

I felt some tragedy of the vulnerable in their own environment and longed to save each one. I wanted to see them thrive as they were, wild and free, in a perfectly-adapted landscape. All of my hope for them swelled as my eyes registered one, or many, and I turned the wheel or braked accordingly. I probably swerved away from nearly 200 rabbits.

In the end, I was grateful to have only hit one.

~ ~ ~

They faded out the way they came in. A full flush, to a trickle, to none. It was hard to even grasp this road now without them. I started to feel like I was floating over a vivid, lucid dream road on top of the known world. At last, I was gliding clearly through now, and I just kept moving. Then, I experienced a new kind of quiet for me. I drove now with a heightened alertness from rabbit-dodging and sweet relief in trusting I would crest this peak. I had that faith in every one of my cells, yet with little evidence to confirm it. What mattered was that I was still going. I felt perfectly calm and awake, relaxed in my body, yet energized in my mind's eye.

I began to breathe into an elated feeling of isolation. I was aware of sleep deprivation - it was maybe 2 or 3 am by now - and I started drawing on a strength I hadn't reached before. I felt I was dreaming, but also vividly wide awake. It was the most alone I had ever been on the road. Literally speaking. Yet, I soon sensed the undeniable presence of something much greater.

That presence and my calm-alert state yielded thoughts that were soothing and reassuring, like the warm, honey voice of love that brought any of us here.

Suddenly, I didn't feel so alone. My whole body tingled with this alive sensation of knowing: something cared immensely. That something held me securely and unwaveringly - not because I was anything unique or special - but simply because I was part of it all. It cared the same way I cared. It felt like my Gramma, yet was somehow more vast and expansive. It included every kind or earnest thing I'd ever seen or experienced.

On a deserted, windy plain in west Texas, I learned I could trust myself to navigate this world. Now, flying over this dark and dream-like mountain pass, I knew I could trust something larger than myself to encourage me, and all of us, toward thriving.

There were all these limited people - parents lacking social courage, headmasters who lie and hide, teachers who choose job security while their students suffer. Young women who run to distant mountains for solace and wisdom-seeking. All of us, limited in our own ways. Yet, together somehow, and greater than any one of us, existed this larger force of caring. I felt it as an expansive mother-love that simply wanted everyone, everything to thrive beyond our imaginations. It wanted me to keep going and also to thrive. *Nothing less, darlin. Nothing less.*

I wept for being alive and having the chance to connect to it at all.

And like it always did, the road held that, too. The joy, relief, and sadness. I felt the gratitude of having come so far, even with still so far yet to go. It all hummed and soothed me once again, and I felt safe. I felt assured of success even inside of a vast unknown. Soon, I could feel the subtle drop of the road, releasing me down with the ease of gravity into a new place. I breathed heavy in relief as a gracious handful of lights twinkled orange-gold in the distance.

I would be there by sunrise.

Major Blessings - The Many Gratitudes

From The Amends Project website, after returning home from Open House in 2018:

Week 28: Giving Thanks

Even when we are tired and depleted beyond measure, when justice is delayed and denied, and when resistance to positive change has caused even more damage . . .
Gratitude. Gratitude . . .

GRATITUDES

to friends who stood beside and behind when facing a wrong was needed to make a right
to the friend who trusted and did what we were taught, and told an adult
to whomever staff heard, and acted, and believed leaders would do right
to the first of those who found me, to concur (#metoo) and thank me for the confrontation at 16
to the school friend who called every week of my subsequent year in exile, to remind me I was not forgotten or even truly lost
to the friend's father, who convinced me to not run away at 17

to the open road, and its surprising graces and medicine
to college professors, who taught me the larger context of social justice and protecting human rights,

Thank You.

to west coast friends and loved ones who supported my long trek east to speak truth & bring a reckoning at 23
to the next round of those who found me, to concur (#metoo) and thank me for this bringing forth
to the boy who sat compelled in the auditorium, who became a man, and found me to speak so clearly in support
to the ways the body strives to protect us and then strengthen us, until it eventually heals us
to every place of sanity, health and love discovered afterward
to the inevitable gathering of molecules of social renewal that force a larger surfacing for healing,

Thank You.

to the Boston Globe investigative reporters, Mitchell Garabedian, and yes, all that the internet makes possible
to the creators & advancers of Restorative Justice
to Saroeum Phoung and decades of courage & dedication
to the women of the Center for Restorative Justice at Suffolk, for rallying so promptly and beautifully to allow this first new step
to brilliantly clear and supportive friends on the west coast,
to enduring, stalwart friends who listen and show up and listen and show up
to mothers who keep all sorts of important documents tucked away
to all mothers who stand up and speak up,

Thank You.

to Rick Sobey and Jim Campinini at the Lowell Sun
to the thousands of viewers, sharers and petition signers

to the next round of those who found me, to concur and thank me for speaking so loudly
to everyone who has bravely endured silencing or institutional abuse alone
to the brilliant, clear, enlightened alumni advisor for hours & hours of insightful bolstering and guidance
to west coast alumni travelers and defenders of justice
to agitators and circulators and vocal old friends of all kinds
to so many alumni – and even friends of alumni – for lending voice and leverage
to Abby Yanow for generous, skillful advising
to coordinators of the Somerville, MA Green Room for support above and beyond
to deeply loyal, supportive, loving west coast friends
to Marci Hamilton, Child USA, Mass Kids, S.E.S.A.M.E, Jane Doe, Shael Norris, Safe Bae, Massachusetts & New Hampshire legislators, progressive media and numerous professors, advocates and advisors around the country
to Justine Finn of the Relation-Shift Project at Harvard Innovation Lab
to Mike Rinaldi, and a model of endurance that heals
to the continuous waves of those who find me to concur/confirm and thank me
to all the donors of the **GoFundMe page**
to the synchronicity of encountering profound generosity while in pursuit of justice,

Thank You.

to the organizers of **All Survivors Day** and the courage to not waver in the face of brute force
to all weavers of resources and gifts in so many forms, to allow me to simply keep going
to the woman with shaky hands who registered me at Lawrence Academy Open House
to Jamie Baker, for profound humanity, integrity and fortitude amidst the surrounding confusion & fear
to every Groton, Massachusetts business that willingly, eagerly displayed The

Amends Project information so prominently
to every moment of shift in the hearts of Lawrence Academy faculty, staff, donors and trustees – away from lockdown/fear – toward the warm hopefulness of possibility
to every moment of aligned courage, in those unseen to me
to the promise of **The Justice CORPS**, and a time when institutional cover-up of child abuse is no longer
to the latent goodness in Steve Hahn
to the latent goodness in Dan Scheibe
to the latent goodness in Paul Lannon
to the latent goodness in Bruce MacNeil
to the willingness of every strong and humane adult around this issue, to stand and speak and act,
Thank You.
Thank You.
Thank You.

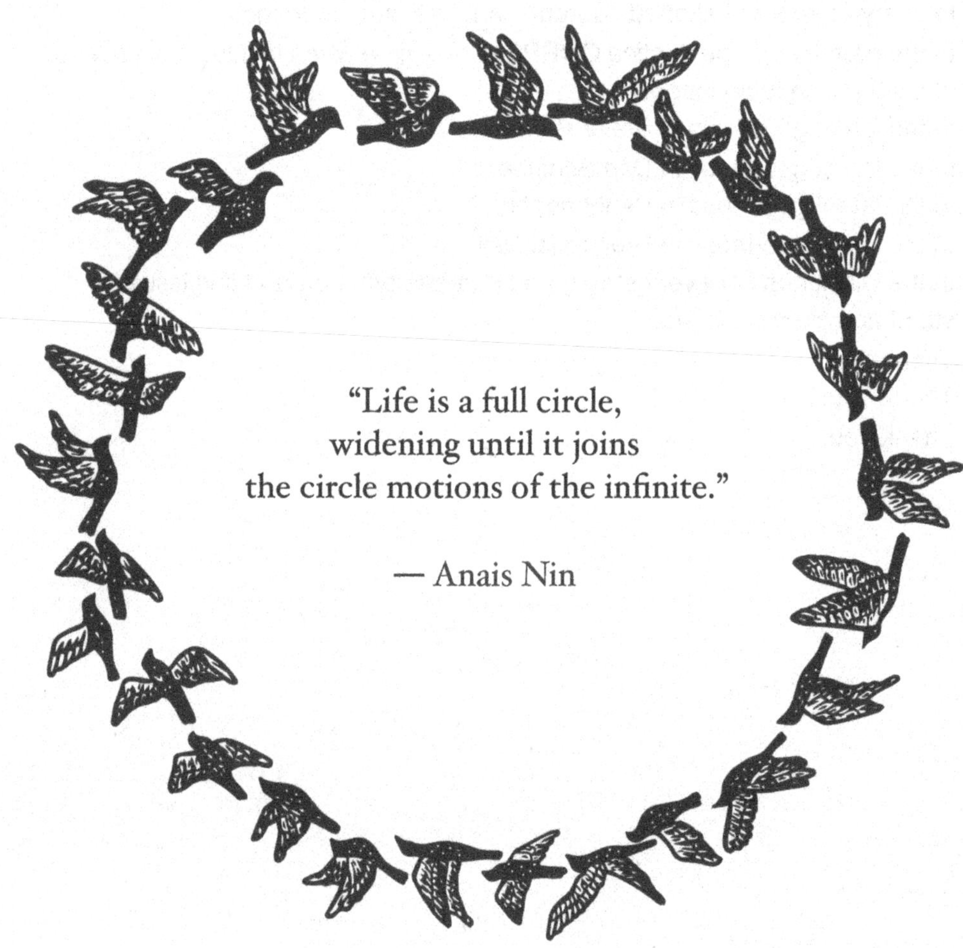

"Life is a full circle,
widening until it joins
the circle motions of the infinite."

— Anais Nin

Taking Action - 2020 & Beyond

February 12, 2020

Dear Massachusetts State Representatives,

I am writing today as a Massachusetts-born advocate and concerned citizen on a mission.

According to the Internal Revenue Service, IRS, charitable nonprofit organizations must abide by two important clauses:

1. the purpose of preventing cruelty to children; and
2. that no private interest may benefit by its operation

Right now, in the United States, private "nonprofit" high schools are concealing child abuse on their campuses, while high-earning headmasters and staff are benefiting from the systematic silencing of children and families.

We need your help to reconcile these core conflicts of interest and purpose in Massachusetts.

When the Boston Globe released their Spotlight Investigation into Boarding Schools in 2016, the country was rattled by the disturbing reality. An alarmingly high number of "respectable" organizations, many federally registered 501(c)3 nonprofits, were overseeing the unthinkable, and causing further damage by their efforts to conceal the truth.

It is time to bring about change, first on the state, and eventually, the Federal level. I ask you to be the leaders that Massachusetts residents elected you to be, and take steps to remedy this situation immediately. Specifically, I reach out today as President of The Amends Project, a nonprofit with the mission to "mend the loophole that has allowed for the cover up of child abuse at independent schools". The Amends Project is one of 79 local and national organizations working on a Federal Initiative to protect the wellbeing of children, and heal the fractures in civic society.

Sister Organizations to this Federal Initiative include the #MeToo Movement, Child USA, RAINN, The US Human Rights Network, MassKids and so many more. We are grateful to SNAP, the Survivors Network of those Abused by Priests, for leading this effort and creating a careful List of Compiled Asks, for changes on the federal level. With Boston at the heart of so many of these painfully revealed stories, I implore you as a Massachusetts Representative to act quickly.

The Ask

The measure of any great unveiling is the power of the awakening that follows. This moment now calls for concrete action, to give positive momentum to the urgency before us. We ask you to:

"Create and champion legislation that would remove nonprofit status of any institution that has failed to act in the best interest of children or vulnerable adults."

Fiscal Responsibility

On the fiscal level, a government cannot justify granting tax-exempt status and benefits to organizations where harms to its members cost our country's healthcare infrastructure untold amounts each year. The national investment in tax incentives is meant to protect the Commonwealth. The costs of such harms must be borne by those failing to protect their members, and not by the people of Massachusetts or America as a whole.

Conflict of Interest & Purpose

To review the current IRS language for charitable nonprofits:

"The exempt purposes set forth in Internal Revenue Code section 501(c)(3) are charitable, religious, educational, scientific, literary, testing for public safety, fostering national or international amateur sports competition, and the prevention of cruelty to children or animals."

The disqualifying language already exists in current legal parlance. Let it be restated here, in no uncertain terms: retaliation, defamation and/or the silencing of young people and families in the wake of abuse is cruelty to children.

The conflict lies in nonprofit, private schools proclaiming a mission to enhance the wellbeing of children, while simultaneously carrying out institutional abuse.

Benefitting Private Interests, "May Not Inure"

Federal Law also clearly states that:

"A section 501(c)(3) organization must not be organized or operated for the benefit of private interests, such as the creator or the creator's family, shareholders of the organization, other designated individuals, or persons controlled directly or indirectly by such private interests.

No part of the net earnings of a section 501(c)(3) organization may inure to the benefit of any private shareholder or individual. A private shareholder or individual is a person having a personal and private interest in the activities of the organization."

When a headmaster, trustee or other official seeks to protect his or her position at the expense of a student or organization member, they are directly benefitting their own private interests. Poignantly, the definition of the verb ***inure*** is, "*to habituate to something undesirable, especially by prolonged subjection*". Our country has been too long subjected to the idea that a corrupted few will benefit at the expense of a vulnerable many.

The Role of Title IX & Exemptions

Title IX is the Federal Law prohibiting discrimination on the basis of sex in education programs or activities that receive federal funding. Currently, a number of private school decision-makers enjoy exemption from Title IX, while leaving their students vulnerable to unequal protections under the law.

To review, this means that certain private, nonprofit schools in Massachusetts are exempt from taxation via their charitable status, and also exempt from upholding ethical standards in the treatment of their members under Title IX. Please consider for a moment, the risks this combination holds, and our obligations to our fellow citizens, equally deserving of justice.

Until these organizations can come into a higher level of compliance for ethical handling, it is imperative that we take a first step towards de-incentivizing abuse and corruption by removing tax-exempt status from organizations failing to protect children and vulnerable adults.

The First Small Step

While a problem of this size can often feel overwhelming, this specific ask - with all of its positive implications - is a simple, practice way to enact positive change now. We are trusting in you to take this first, small step.

Removing nonprofit status from Massachusetts-based organizations that fail to act in the best interest of children sends a message to the country that citizens of the state expect more from their charitable, nonprofit organizations. If Massachusetts led the way in revealing disturbing institutional inner-workings, it is only right that you, as representatives, now lead the way in proudly taking steps toward repairing the problem, once and for all.

As a leading member in a network of dedicated human rights organizations, I offer you this language, and the opportunity, to stand with us in protecting human rights and dignity for all.

Thank You.

Sincerely,

Vanessa Osage

Vanessa Osage
President, The Amends Project
https://theamendsproject.com

In October 2020, Vanessa Osage will be presenting The Justice CORPS Initiative at the Association of Title IX Administrators, ATIXA, East Coast Conference in Philadelphia, PA (now available remotely).

She continues to apply for presenting The Justice CORPS Initiative at the National Association of Independent Schools, NAIS, People of Color Conference. This year's theme is *New Decade, New Destinies: Challenging Self, Changing Systems and Choosing Justice*. The conference will be held remotely, because of the Coronavirus pandemic.

During the four months of Washington state "stay-at-home" orders, while writing this book, two more former classmates contacted Vanessa Osage about institutional child abuse: one from Notre Dame Academy in Tyngsboro, Massachusetts and Bishop Guertin in Nashua, New Hampshire; and one to offer support to her, upon receiving news of another lawsuit at Lawrence Academy of Groton, Massachusetts.

She has applied to be a speaker with Humanities Washington's Speakers Bureau, traveling the state to lead an interactive workshop called, *Speak Truth to Power*, from 2021-2022.

Vanessa Osage is seeking angel investors to fund The Justice CORPS for a pilot run at two schools, from anywhere in the country, for the 2021-2022 school year.

Lawrence Academy headmaster and Board of Trustees are still yet to acknowledge the cover up or to settle with Ms. Osage out of court.

Ancient Parable

According to an ancient parable,
a king quarrels with his son and in a fit of rage,
exiles his son from the kingdom.
After a number of years,
the king's heart softens,
and he sends his ministers to find his son
and ask him to come home.

But, the young man resists the invitation.
He feels too bitter, too hurt to return.
When the ministers present the sad news to the king,
he sends them out with a new message.
"Return as far as you can,
and I will come the rest of the way
to meet you."

Choose Your Own Ending

To add your story to an anonymous online catalogue of accounts, visit: http://theamendsproject.com/add-your-story/

To support success of The Justice CORPS Initiative, please visit: https://theamendsproject.com/support-the-movement/

For professional coaching, consulting, or education with Vanessa Osage, & to book speaking engagements, visit: www.loveandtruthrising.org

To encourage Lawrence Academy of Groton, Massachusetts school leaders to admit, apologize, and amend, email:
Headmaster Daniel Scheibe, dscheibe@lacademy.edu
Board of Trustees Member Bruce MacNeil, macneiltrustee@lacademy.edu
Attorney Paul Lannon, paul.lannon@hklaw.com

To apply for early participation in The Justice CORPS pilot program, and receive a documentary film chronicling your school's experience, visit: http://theamendsproject.com/apply-the-justice-corps/

www.vanessaosage.com

www.theamendsproject.com

Value & Appreciation

I've offered my voice at the crest of an immense wave of love, passion, support, encouragement and visionary social courage. Every one of these people has played a valuable role in uplifting this moment. I give each of you my profound gratitude and appreciation.

~ ~ ~

The Changemakers Alliance, Millworks Co-Housing, Rooted Emerging contributors, The Amends Project Advisors, Justine Finn, Abby Yanow, Mike Rinaldi, Shael Norris, Leah Jarkko, Jamie Baker, Brian Feigenbaum, Sybil Johnson, Naomi Siegel, Mary Tully, Nicole Whitney, Kira Swanson & family, Alderney Sisu, Anu Byal, Terri Wilde, Peg Davies, Marjorie Leone, Nicole Hurtibise, Lisa Dailey of Sidekick Press, Mary Knight, Kathy Bastow, Catriona Munro & family, Carrie Bishop-Cruz, Liz Darrow, Anni Kamola, Greg Estes, Dr. Julia Hipp, Beth Schultz, Blake Goldsworthy, Kirk Murphy, Nick Nordquist, The Van Worden Family, The Jarkko Family, Rhea Tamanakis, Cole Melendy, Isaiah Mendehlson Meyer, Laura Mendelsohn Meyer, Holly Johnson, Sollis Edmond Hale, Utina Psaltis, Jerry Mead, Erin Taff, Matt Lamb, Kip Bordelon, Trevor Smith, Greg Sheehan, Damon Jespersen, Noah Elder, Matt Patrick, Avital Melnicker, Alex Hayes, Marguerite Bryant, Richard Bissell, Jennifer Cohen & family, Sue Richardson & family, Rachel Billingsly, David Koshinz, Sarah Clarke, Esther Kathryn

McRill, Edward Fatjo, Saroeum Phoung, Tiffany Dedeaux, Nicki Lang, Joan Elk, Dustin & Julia Whitney, James Dunstone, Jenna Bean Veatch, Stephanie Manzo, Rachael Mueller, Kathy Bastow, Lisa Tenney, Charlie Eagle, Judi Horvath, Bree Eagle, Holly Johnson, Poppi's Anatolia, Caroline Boyes-Watson, The Center for Restorative Justice at Suffolk University, Mitchell Garabedian, Rick Sobey, Zach Hiner, Tim Lennon, SNAP, The Sexual Health Advocates Group, SHAG, Myra McGovern, Donna Orem, Peter Upham, The Association of Boarding Schools, TABS, The National Association of Independent Schools, NAIS, The Association of Title IX Administrators, ATIXA, all of my clients, all the families served, every school who has hired me as a teacher or guest speaker, every petition-signer, every parent or alumni who reached out, everyone who cheers this on out of view from me, Chris Testa & Cadence Osage Testa

Thank You

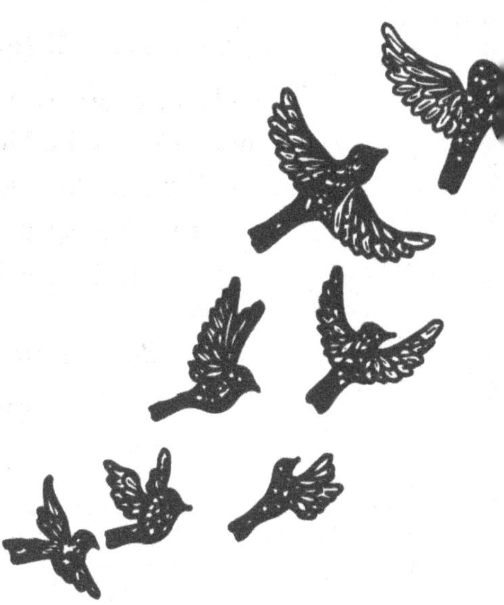

Vanessa Osage is a tell-it-like-it-is east-coaster and a visionary west coaster. Her writing has appeared in Circles on the Mountain, The Confluence Journal, ICF World, Role Reboot & more. She was a small-town newspaper reporter, once upon a time. She lives in Bellingham, Washington.

Stay informed of upcoming books at:

vanessaosage.com

@vanessaosage

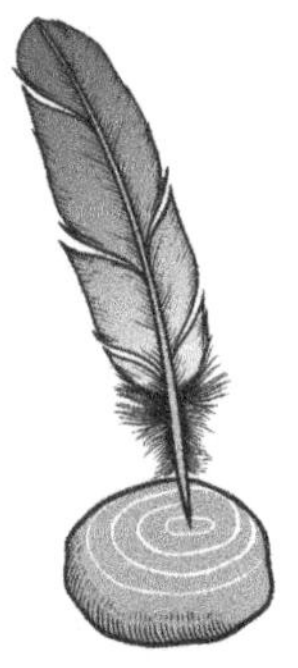

Stone & Feather Press

publishes stories that may otherwise be forgotten. We advance human, civil, and environmental rights by promoting justice through powerful storytelling.

This title is also available as an audiobook at

stoneandfeatherpress.com